How to Pleasurably Stop Smoking

D0317220

80003420402

ALSO BY JIM ANDREWS

vispo.com

How to *Pleasurably* Stop Smoking

Jim Andrews

vispo.com, Vancouver

2016

Copyright © 2016 by Jim Andrews
Vispo.com publishing
vispo.com

All rights reserved. This book or any portion thereof may not be reproduced or used in any manner whatsoever without the express written permission of the publisher except for the use of brief quotations in a book review or scholarly journal.

Library and Archives Canada Cataloguing in Publication Data

Andrews, Jim 1959—
　　How to Pleasurably Stop Smoking / Jim Andrews
ISBN: 978-0-9949531-0-0

Second edition

Cover images

- "Girl With a Cigarette" is an 1850 painting by Petr Zabolotskiy (1803-1866). Public domain image: commons.wikimedia.org/wiki/File:1850_Zabolotskiy_Girl_with_a_cigarette_anagoria.JPG

- George Arents Collection, The New York Public Library. "Raleigh's first pipe in England" The New York Public Library Digital Collections. digitalcollections.nypl.org/items/510d47dc-89c5-a3d9-e040-e00a18064a99

- "God L, Palenque, Temple of the Cross" is an image of a Mayan deity, associated with trade, smoking a cigar. Public domain image: https://en.wikipedia.org/wiki/God_L . Photo by Peter Isoltalo.

- Freud by Max Halberstadt, 1921. Public domain image: commons.wikimedia.org/wiki/File:Sigmund_Freud_LIFE.jpg

Images in book

- Flammarion engraving. Public domain image: en.wikipedia.org/wiki/Flammarion_engraving

For my parents Evelyn and Dick

and my mom's sisters Elinor and Georgie

Northamptonshire Libraries & Informaton Services BB	
Askews & Holts	

Contents

Acknowledgments

Thanks to my wife Natalie Funk for feedback on the manuscript as I was writing it. You almost invariably identified the problems and offered valuable advice on them. But you also were articulate about what you liked. This was something we did together, for which I am grateful. Your support strengthened this book as it warms and strengthens me, Natalie.

Thanks also to Adeena Karasick for permission to quote her. But, also, thanks for being the first smoker to allow me to talk with you as you read the book and then talked with you about your changing perspective on smoking and stopping smoking. This subsequent edition is much better because of our conversations. Especially the emphasis on breath and breathing, a concern and interest we share as poets and vocal performers.

1 - How to Prepare to Stop Smoking

When should you read this book? What are the conditions required for you to use it successfully? If you're ready to stop smoking, the book will take you to the point where you do indeed stop and it will help you make it permanent.

The main goal is for you to stop successfully by the time you finish reading the book, but not everybody is at that stage—yet. If you're not ready to stop smoking by the end of the book, the book will nonetheless show you what you need to reach the point where you *are* ready to stop, and it will start you on that road by changing your perspective on smoking—and on stopping smoking. And it will give you some tools to start using now that will help you to stop, when you're ready to stop.

You can smoke as you read this book, if you haven't yet stopped smoking. By the time you're finished the book, if we're on schedule, you will have no desire to smoke.

What I need you to commit to, for you to use this book successfully, is this: if, when you finish the book, you no longer desire to smoke— that is, you're not experiencing urges to smoke—you have to be willing to stop smoking. That isn't asking much of you because if you have no urges to smoke, no desire to smoke, then you will almost certainly *very gladly* stop smoking.

If you're still experiencing urges to smoke, after you've finished the book, you may not be ready to stop smoking yet.

It isn't as though this book will work once and only once. The approach this book takes to stopping smoking—namely, first and foremost helping you get rid of the desire to smoke—is always your first and best option in stopping smoking. But effectively dismantling the illusions that support your desire to smoke—permanently—is the final stage of stopping smoking. If you're not there yet and won't be for a while, you need the tools to get there. The book provides those tools.

In short, the book puts you on the road to stopping smoking. Whether you are at the end of that road or the beginning, it helps you understand the territory and find your way to a successful eventual conclusion. The book is especially rewarding—even exciting—if you are indeed ready to stop.

Stopping smoking permanently is the best smoking-related experience of all. Every day after you've stopped, you're happy to be a non-smoker, you're deservedly proud of having gotten to that point in your life, you see your life is much better without smoking and you also enjoy life much more without smoking. Also, the process of stopping smoking, contrary to popular opinion, should be a *rewarding experience*—one of the *best* experiences of your life.

You don't need to be on holidays. You don't even need to want to stop smoking right now. You just need to want to stop smoking permanently; and you should want to know how to pleasurably stop smoking.

That's the road ahead. Read on if you dare.

2 - The Program in a Nutshell

This book is for those who want to stop smoking, those who have stopped but find that they still want to smoke, and those who think about issues of tobacco, smoking, and addiction.

The problem with many approaches to stopping smoking is that they require too much willpower. You want to smoke but have to continually resist your desire to smoke. Most people eventually give in to their desire.

What we're going to do is different. It doesn't require so much willpower. Here's the program. We're going to get rid of your desire to smoke. Obviously it wouldn't be hard to stop if you had no desire to smoke. You're going to get to that point and learn how to retain your lack of desire to smoke. So that it's permanent. That's the program in a nutshell.

Addiction to nicotine has two fundamental components: the physical and psychological addictions. Many people find it surprising to learn that the psychological component of the addiction is the hardest issue to successfully address. Getting rid of your desire to smoke is mainly a matter of dismantling the psychological addiction.

Nicotine addiction is like an iceberg: there's the part you see and the part you don't. The part you don't see is the biggest part: the psychological addiction. The physical addiction is the visible part.

The physical addiction is over in less than a week. Also, the physical sensation of withdrawal is subtle, unlike the withdrawal symptoms from alcohol or heroin. The sensation of nicotine withdrawal is of light-headedness and mild hunger. What makes stopping smoking difficult is the way that the sensation of hunger for nicotine gets *amplified* into *urges* by the psychological addiction.

When we dismantle the psychological addiction, we unplug the *amplifier*. In the week after you stop, while the physical addiction is still present, rather than experiencing *urges* to smoke, you experience the actual *physical sensation* of nicotine withdrawal, which is much easier to deal with. You don't experience the urgency associated with urges because you will have no desire to smoke. All you will experience is something like occasional mild hunger, and this sensation will pass. As the physical dependence disappears over the course of a week, even that mild hunger-like sensation will cease permanently.

It's like the difference between an appointment with the Wizard of Oz when he is right in front of you versus when he is hiding behind the facade with amplifiers, fire and brimstone. The amplifiers, fire and brimstone make him seem more powerful, fearful, and persuasive than he is. He's much easier to deal with without the amplifiers.

Some people experience stopping smoking as torturous. Because they are trying to stop doing something they desperately want to do. The way you're going to do it, there is no torture or desperation. To the contrary, stopping should be *one of the best experiences of your life*. It's certainly the top smoking-related experience! Smoking is ho-hum compared with stopping smoking, if done right.

You see more clearly. You see that what kept you smoking is gone. You don't desire it anymore. You're free of it. Those who know what it's like to be a slave to a substance know how much they'd like to be free of it. Stopping smoking successfully is an experience of gaining self-knowledge and freedom. Freedom that requires defending, but real freedom. Freedom from the desire to smoke and, with that freedom, freedom also from smoking.

With that freedom goes a need to experience its joy and satisfaction. Rejoicing in your freedom from addiction helps you stay free. Because if you can really *feel that joy and satisfaction* every day, when you call on it, that helps you deal with what is left of the urge to smoke after the amplifier is unplugged. Because you appreciate what you have. You can feel it. You think 'Would I rather have a cigarette or feel what I am feeling now?' If you can feel the joy you have earned, you'd rather feel that joy. If you can feel the pleasure of breathing fresh air, you can appreciate it and cherish it.

When you see the nature and power of the illusions that have kept you smoking until now, you glimpse the veil of tears, the fabric of this life. You see how powerful illusions can be. You come to a deeper *understanding and appreciation* of yourself and the world.

The experience of stopping smoking is thought to be hellish. It is if you retain the desire to smoke. But if you have no desire to smoke, it's as easy as it is to resist staring at the sun.

That's where we're going by the end of the book. Some get there and some don't. If it doesn't work for you, don't despair. Many people stop smoking several times before it's permanent. You eventually succeed. But each time you try is *necessary* in your journey; you learn important things about yourself and your addiction in the process. Understanding why you continue to smoke is crucial; so is being able to deal with the fictitious stories you tell yourself to start smoking again.

You might think the goal is to stop smoking. But that happens automatically if you meet a different goal. The goal is to *understand why you continue to smoke* and therefore understand what benefits you think smoking gives you. You'll come to understand that smoking doesn't give you *any* of those things.

The other thing you need to do is end the romance with smoking. To dismantle your psychological addiction to smoking, you free your *head* of illusions about smoking and your *heart* of the romance with smoking.

One of the things we'll look at in the last part of the book is the 9,000 year history of smoking. From tobacco shamanism in the Americas through the European and, not long after that, global adoption of tobacco starting in the 1500s. Why look at that history? So much has changed since then. Even the tobacco is different—it used to be hallucinogenic, believe it or not. And we don't use it religiously, unlike many of the indigenous peoples of the Americas. What of that history is relevant to your desire to stop smoking now?

So much has changed but the fundamental dynamic has not. For thousands of years, people have ascribed medicinal and other powers to tobacco and smoking that they don't actually have. Smoking has always supplied a convincing illusion of offering important benefits.

Getting to the bottom of those very old illusions, understanding them clearly—through the ages and across vastly different cultures—is crucial.

What do we see through those convincing smoky illusions? Do we see the menacing grin of Tezcatlipoca, Aztec god of tobacco commanding us beyond our ability to resist? Not so much. We see *ourselves*, our naked, vulnerable, human frailty and need for reassurance and assistance in a world we do not command. It's an old story of our desire for help.

3 - The Little Monster and the Big Monster

An addiction is not the same as a habit. Habits are easily broken. I eat certain things in my breakfast. I could and sometimes do eat something else for breakfast or don't have any at all. Another habit I have is following a certain route when I go for a jog. I could easily change that route if I felt I needed to. *Habits* are not normally *compulsive*; they're easily changed or dropped.

An addiction is *compulsive* behavior that addicts persist in even in the face of negative consequences. An addiction is a habit that addicts feel unwilling and unable to stop even when faced with negative consequences.

Overeating can be an addiction but *eating*, per se, is not an addiction because there are no negative consequences to continuing to eat normally; we need to eat to survive but, with addictions, the compulsion to continue is not caused by a biological necessity but, primarily, a psychological dependence on the perceived (but illusory) contribution of the behavior to our well-being.

Addicts are convinced of the value of the behavior; they feel it gives them something they need. They do truly need what they *think* the addiction gives them, but the addiction doesn't supply it at all. They supply it themselves. They think that going without what they're addicted to would result in a quality of life that would barely be worth living, but eventually the addiction itself reduces the quality of their life drastically.

There may be a physical addiction involved, such as in smoking, heroin, cocaine, alcohol, coffee and other substances where unpleasant physical withdrawal symptoms occur.

But an addiction *does not require a substance*. Gambling is clearly a terrible addiction for some people. They lose all their money and gamble away money they don't have. They don't stop until they aren't allowed to gamble anymore. It ruins families. It can *definitely* be compulsive behavior that the gambler persists in even in the face of *extremely* negative consequences.

People can be addicted to relationships that are over. So that the other person gets a restraining order. But they still feel compelled to see the other person. Stalkers go to prison.

People can be addicted to stealing (kleptomania) or setting fires (pyromania). High-risk compulsive behavior is not unknown in extreme sports such as wingsuit base jumping. One type of addiction is thrill seeking.

People can be addicted to shopping, playing video games, sex, viewing pornography, working, exercising, seeking pain, cutting themselves, the Internet...on and on. Addiction is compulsive behavior that the addict persists in even in the face of negative consequences. Even when they want to stop, they feel powerless to do so.

The idea that addiction is all about the influence of a substance on our mind and body is mistaken. Addictive substances *do* influence our body and mind. But, as we have seen, there exist addictions such as gambling that exhibit all the hallmarks of addiction *except there is no substance involved*. They can be just as destructive as addictions that have a physical component.

This highlights the importance of the psychological aspect of addiction. Addictions aren't necessarily to substances but they *always* involve psychological dependence. It's relatively easy to deal with the physical aspect of addiction *if the psychological dependence is dismantled*. In the case of smoking, the physical addiction is much less powerful than it's widely misunderstood to be. Withdrawal symptoms from nicotine feel like mild hunger together with slight light-headedness. When you stop smoking, they last about a week. Allen Carr called the physical symptoms "the little monster".

"The big monster" is the psychological dependence. Or, as he called it, the "brainwashing". *Our belief* that smoking is making an important contribution to our well-being, to our quality of life, to our desire to enjoy life, is the main source of our compulsion to smoke. Even if there is biochemistry at work—even in addictions like gambling, where there is no physical substance consumed—that creates urges, as some researchers maintain is the case, those urges are predicated on our belief that the object of the addiction is doing something very special for us. Identifying what those special things are we seek through the addiction, and then also understanding that the addiction doesn't give them to us, is very helpful in dispelling the illusion the addiction requires to maintain its hold on us.

The physical addiction is a regular prompter of our compulsion.

Every time we have a cigarette, that helps create physical withdrawal symptoms in the future. The physical withdrawal symptoms prompt us to feel the urge to smoke. So do things like anxiety, fear, and stress.

What is the urge to smoke if it isn't simply physical hunger for nicotine? The urge to smoke is an *amplification* of the mild hunger sensation of the physical addiction. What amplifies it? The psychological dependence amplifies it. How does the psychological dependence amplify it?

Often smokers smoke when they feel anxiety about something. Sometimes the anxiety is caused simply by nicotine withdrawal but at other times the anxiety has some other cause. The greater the anxiety, fear, sadness, sorrow—or even celebratory emotion—the greater the desire for a cigarette. In other words, the anxiety/stress/emotion amplifies the mild hunger of the physical addiction into an urge. The greater the anxiety, the stronger the urge. Without the anxiety, there would only be the mild hunger of the physical addiction. The anxiety amplifies the mild hunger of the physical addiction into an urge. The urge is sometimes perceived as a purely physical consequence of the physical dependence but, really, the strength of the urge is proportional to the anxiety or emotion. We use smoking as a way to reduce or cope with stress, anxiety, worry, and anything else we would like relief from such as work. Smoking is self-medication for such things. It's medication that doesn't actually work, but it provides a good illusion that it works.

Soothing the urge to smoke by smoking—does this alleviate the anxiety? It temporarily alleviates the anxiety caused by the physical withdrawal symptoms, but it doesn't do much for the anxiety caused by something other than smoking. People experience *less* anxiety *after they stop smoking* because smoking causes far more anxiety than it alleviates.

Sometimes smokers smoke to concentrate on what they want to think about—or to forget about something. The urge is as strong as their desire to concentrate (or forget). In this case, excitement or dread amplifies the desire.

Just as one can be addicted to all sorts of different things, the urge to smoke can be an urge for a variety of things. Mostly urges to smoke are made of whatever anxiety, fear, apprehension, desire, excitement, sadness, etc you are feeling at the moment. Urges are made of your emotions and desires. It's important that you think about and get a handle on the different forms of your urge to smoke and, more particularly, the ones that are most important to you. So that you can dismantle your amplifier.

For thrill seekers, it can be sublimated sexuality. If you've ever seen a woman smoke a cigarette with the deliberation of noir, you've seen how smoking can convey smoldering sexuality. The urge to smoke is conveyed as an urge for the intoxication of romance, of sex, of adventure, of the thrilling.

Other people (or the same people at a different time) reach for a cigarette like it's a life preserver on choppy seas. They seek calming. They're wound up—at least in part because of nicotine withdrawal— but just generally wound up, also, in their lives, so the urge to smoke is associated with the calming of anxiety, of stress, and of relaxation.

To watch philosophical smokers smoke, you half expect to see their smoke imbued with visual, kinetic poetry. The urge to smoke, for them, is toward concentration and intellectual meditation.

Smoking is multi-functional. We use it to 'help' and medicate ourselves in various ways. These are tailored to the individual's particular needs, fears, insecurities, and desires, to some extent. But there is not an infinity of significantly different configurations; the configurations are relatively few in number. What are the needs, fears, insecurities and desires you have that get amplified into urges to smoke?

4 - Some Things Are Best Done Easily

Some things are best done easily: if you make it too hard, you're not doing it right. Stopping smoking is one of those things. It's considered to be incredibly hard to do—and *it is* if you go about it the wrong way. If you don't get rid of the *desire to smoke*, then you end up Jonesing for a cigarette. That's a hard way to stop. But if you get rid of the desire to smoke, then it doesn't take any more willpower than the amount required to refrain from jumping off a tall building. Most people don't have a problem refraining from jumping off tall buildings.

Another example of something that is best done easily is asking someone out on a date. People tie themselves into knots about it. Because they're terrified of being rejected. Fear creates a wall, though, that makes it likely the person will say no. The answer to whether someone wants to go out with you depends on whether you can enjoy each others' company and have a good time together. *You* also need to know the answer to that question. You both find that out *during the very time you might end up asking them out*. That should be a fun occasion of communication between you. If it is, then you'll both probably want to go out together. If it isn't, then at least one of you won't want to repeat the experience. Asking someone out should be easy in the sense that if there is a spark between the two of you, asking the other person out will not be a terrifying ordeal but an exciting thing pleasantly anticipated by both people. If it's something you want to enjoy and really want to explore, it will probably go well. If it's a terrifying ordeal, the other person will probably not be attracted. It should be easy in the sense that it isn't a terrifying ordeal but, instead, is a confirmation that you both already feel a spark. It's exciting to ask someone out if there's a real connection.

Performing as an actor or poet/storyteller or playing competitive sports are also examples of things that are best done easily. If fear gets the best of you and you can't enjoy the performance or the game/competition, then you are likely to do poorly. You need to be relaxed and aware. It should be easy in the sense that it's not a terrifying ordeal but an exciting, real adventure of the physical or mental variety—or both. You just do with joy and intensity what you've been practicing for a long time. All the practice has made it easy—as long as fear doesn't get in the way. It's rewarding and fun if fear doesn't dominate the picture.

These things that are best done easily have something else in common: if fear rules the day, they become excruciatingly difficult and bound to fail. There isn't anyone who has ever lived who hasn't been terrified of being rejected at some time. Everyone knows exactly what that feels like. And there isn't a performer who hasn't been terrified of performing in front of an audience, or an athlete who hasn't choked, at some point, out of fear. Just like there isn't a smoker who hasn't been afraid of stopping smoking. It's just part of the experience. A part that you eventually learn to get beyond.

Getting rid of that fear is an interesting, empowering experience which you are going to experience. Now or later. Might as well be now. That fear is important to how the amplifier amplifies the weak twitch of physical addiction into urges for cigarettes. Without that fear, you're almost free.

How does fear sometimes rule when people want to stop smoking? Smokers are afraid that they will have to give up things they enjoy, and that they won't be able to enjoy life like they did when they smoked. But the way we're going to do it, you will not only enjoy life *more* when you stop smoking—you will enjoy the process of stopping smoking, also. It won't be an excruciating experience of deprivation but an enriching experience that will deprive you of *nothing* that you enjoy.

Moreover, this is best done easily, not as something that is difficult. When I hear about the easy way to do anything, I am suspicious. Some things are just plain difficult. There is no easy way to program computers and anyone who says there is is selling snake oil.

But stopping smoking is not like that. Why not? Smoking *should be and is* easy to stop because the only things it has going for it are your belief that it gives you something you need, and your romance with it. You think that smoking gives you something you really value. This book is all about coming to realize it doesn't. This book is all about coming to a solid realization that the idea that smoking gives you anything you need or value or desire or want *is an illusion*. That is all smoking has going for it: your belief in the illusion that you need and want it. Once you disabuse yourself of that illusion, *you don't want it or need it anymore*. That's how you get rid of the desire to smoke.

That's the nature of psychological addiction. It involves an illusion that the object of the addiction (smoking, in this case) gives you something you need. Once that illusion is removed, you realize you don't need or want it.

It's like the illusion of a 'magic' trick. Once you understand how the trick works, it no long er has any power over you. It's so completely finished, you're so over it that it just isn't ever going to work on you again.

Stopping smoking *should be and is* easy if you go about it the right way, which is how you're going to do it.

5 - Relation to Allen Carr's Book

According to Allen Carr in his book *The Easy Way to Stop Smoking*, the biggest problem for smokers to overcome is brainwashing or, in other words, illusions. It's fascinating that at the core of the problem is brainwashing/illusion. Most people think of chemical addiction as being at the core of the problem. And it is—but it's not the hardest part of the problem; the physical addiction, according to Carr and also according to my own experience, is much less powerful than one's illusions, one's brainwashing.

Carr saw this very clearly. He was an independent thinker. Mind you, it took him 35 years to arrive there. Better late than never! I wasn't much faster; I smoked for 30 years. I'm hoping to help you improve significantly on that! Carr doesn't explore a lot of the implications of his insights except insofar as they help the reader stop smoking. Although he did write other books on how to deal with other addictions such as drinking and over-eating; he did see his ideas as being more broadly applicable than solely to stopping smoking. But he focused on being a therapist, not a theoretician.

Reading Carr's book has been the start of a welcome liberation for me not only from smoking but in understanding the power of illusions. And in understanding why we come to embrace and believe illusions that only convince those who want to believe them.

Carr wasn't a writer, initially. He was an accountant before he started treating smokers. But his books have renewed and restored my faith in the transformative possibilities books offer us. That a book can be such a strong help in stopping smoking is inspiring.

What I've tried to do is write a book that can be read on its own but goes well with a reading of Allen Carr's book. Carr's book endeavors to turn you into a non-smoker before you finish reading his book. What audacity! What a claim! But it's brilliant. And it's worked for millions of people. It's an amazing accomplishment, both for Carr and for the reader. Yet it unfolds, for the reader, without any great effort. It truly is the easy way to stop smoking. You read the book with engagement and with an open mind. You deal with your illusions/brainwashing. And then you're free.

Then you have to cultivate and nourish your freedom. You have to be thankful for it. You have to appreciate it. You have to rejoice in it. You also need to develop an ability to observe yourself. When you experience what is left of the desire to smoke, something less than an urge—more like an involuntary twitch or, in the first week, like a mild form of hunger—you need to not get caught up in the sensation but look at it not as a desire to smoke but as a sensation. It isn't an urge anymore. It's a mild sensation that you need to describe to yourself. And know it to be not only something that soon will pass, but also something that will happen less and less frequently.

When I read Carr's book I'd stopped smoking but hadn't understood the psychological nature of the addiction and so, once again, was at risk to start again, as I had several times previously. Reading Carr's book cured me permanently. I will never take it up again. I am as certain of it as I am that 'magic' tricks which have been explained to me will never again appear as magical.

This book is the peanut gallery to Allen Carr's book. This book explores and amplifies points Carr makes in his book. It also explores some of the things that Carr implies but doesn't explore very much. And, finally, the book explores some possibilities that Carr doesn't touch on at all. If you read them both, you'll see they're very different books that help you in related but different ways.

This book will help you to stop smoking permanently. There really isn't anything in this world that I'd like to do more than help you stop smoking, help free you from that affliction. Too many of my nearest and dearest have died from it. This is for them as much as for you and for me.

6 - Why Have You Continued to Smoke?

As Allen Carr observes, the reasons why we should stop smoking are less helpful in our ability to stop smoking than the reasons why we have *continued to smoke*. Just about everyone knows the reasons to stop smoking: it's a killer; it causes innumerable illnesses before it kills you; it steals your health, over time; it's repugnant to non-smokers; you have to do it 200 meters from anywhere; it's a poor example to children; it's expensive; it causes worry and anxiety about what it's doing to you; it's humiliating and disturbing to apparently be powerless to stop doing something you actually would like to stop doing, and so on. No addict worth their salt ever let such considerations stop them. They press on smoking, regardless.

What is really useful, however, to stopping smoking is understanding the reasons why you continue to smoke. Understanding those is, in fact, absolutely crucial. Because once you understand those, you can realize that smoking doesn't give you any of the benefits you have continued to smoke for. And once you realize that, the jig is up. You're free of the urges.

For many people, the reasons why they continue to smoke are the usual ones. They think they need it to concentrate, or they think they need it for relaxation, or stress management. There are a handful of usual reasons.

Tobacco companies appeal to one's insecurities to make addict customers. Some peoples' insecurities run deeper or simply other than the usual reasons. To dismantle your psychological addiction to cigarettes, you don't need to understand the reasons why you continue to smoke at the level of someone who has examined the issue for twenty years in psychotherapy. You simply need to understand that smoking *isn't giving you* the truly important things *you think it's giving you*. You need to get in touch with the real reasons why you continue to smoke. Once you do that, it isn't hard to see that smoking isn't giving you what you think it is.

It's a con game that tobacco companies play with us—one that requires our own participation. We convince ourselves that smoking gives us things it doesn't. That only happens when we want to believe smoking helps make it all better, helps alleviate our fears and insecurities. The greater our fear and insecurity, the more vulnerable we are to the idea that smoking will help us deal with our pain, fear, and anxieties.

The reason why smoking is more prevalent among poor people is because they tend to live in situations that involve more pain, fear, and anxiety. Consequently, they are more vulnerable to the predations of tobacco companies offering false assurances and 'medication' for their suffering.

For most smokers, poor or not, smoking is an attempt at self-medication to alleviate mental pain, fear, and anxiety. It doesn't help. It just makes the situation worse.

Coming to that realization—not in any vague way, but realizing that it doesn't give you yourself the intimate assistance you associate so strongly with it—is crucial to gaining your freedom, to dismantling the psychological addiction, the psychological dependence.

Many people do not require any psychotherapy to come to this level of realization about why they continue to smoke. Others may have to seek help with it. In any case, it's a matter of being able to look at the important reasons, for you, as to why you continue to smoke, whether they are the standard ones or not.

The reasons why we continue to smoke can change over time, also. Youngsters who started smoking to look adult, or because their parents smoke, don't smoke for the same reason twenty years later. The main reason why people continue to smoke is because they are hooked, of course. But they are hooked because they believe illusions, they believe smoking gives them some important things.

What are those things, for you? If you think you need to smoke to get those things like you have them now, you're going to remain hooked. The typical reasons people give about why they continue to smoke are these:

- nicotine addiction
- stress reduction
- relaxation
- something to do with hands
- concentration

- socializing
- enjoyment (they like the taste and the activity)
- fills in time/stops boredom
- keeps weight down

We will discuss each of these in this book.

7 - Don't Give Up

It seemed like whenever I failed at something, my dad would say to me "If at first you don't succeed, try try again." It was annoying to hear it so much! Annoying, but my father's help and encouragement were nourishing, strengthening—a great help. I would like to offer you the same sort of encouragement concerning your desire to stop smoking.

Most smokers attempt to stop several times before they permanently stop. I did. Each time, I tried to learn something about myself and thought about how to deal with or avoid the situation or reaction that started me smoking again. It's a process of learning about yourself and learning about tobacco addiction to the point where you know what to expect of yourself when you stop. Also, it's a matter of dispelling your illusions about what smoking give you.

The first time I quit was for a woman I was seeing who insisted on it. After we broke up it wasn't long before I was back at it. To be permanent, it needs to be something that you do for yourself, not something you do for somebody else. Not because it requires a lot of willpower that you yourself have to marshal. What you are going to do does not require a lot of willpower.

The first couple of years of a relationship may be enough to help you stop smoking for that time. But, eventually, when the heat is on and maybe you don't have the usual supports, if you haven't dismantled the psychological dependence, it could well assert itself again and cause you to start smoking. Dismantling the psychological dependence gives you a much better chance of stopping permanently.

I can't remember the exact circumstances when I started smoking again, but I do remember the feeling that, not being in the romance with my ex-girlfriend anymore, I had one less big reason to stop smoking and one more to start. I had stopped smoking but I was still under the illusion that smoking had good things to offer me. *That* romance was not over.

I did not value my achievement of stopping smoking enough, either. I didn't even realize that I was still psychologically predisposed to depend on it. I hadn't done much thinking about my addiction. I had used Zyban and the power of love. Which successfully helped me stop for about a year. But without the sort of change in perspective that this book is all about, I was still predisposed, in times of stress, to think that smoking had something to offer.

Later on, when I stopped permanently, I was five years older, had seen my dear father and had seen some other people close to me die of smoking, had gained a lot of weight and was feeling old, for the first time—achy all the time, winded, tired, and unhappy. I'd also tried to stop smoking several more times and had come to grips with the fictions I tell myself to start smoking again. And I'd stopped drinking, for the most part. I could finally value my achievement in stopping smoking appropriately. Not simply because it had been such a long, painful haul—which I really hope you can avoid, because there are higher challenges in life for you besides stopping smoking—but because I knew myself a bit better. And I couldn't lie to myself as easily to start again.

This was all before I read Carr's book. I stopped the hard way. Also, although I had stopped, the romance with smoking was still not really over. I could still occasionally really want one very badly. I was still at high risk of going back to it. Reading Carr's book and thinking about it brought me to the point where it's quite unlikely I will ever start again because, for one thing, I almost never really want a cigarette badly, and on the odd occasion when I do, I can observe that desire from a bit of distance and see it for what it is: not a desire to smoke a cigarette but a desire for something else, an escape from the present situation or a tantalizing elicit pleasure. Or a kind of peace-pipe experience to share with an old friend I smoked and drank with for years. We still get together from time to time and he still smokes. Neither of us drink much anymore, though, which is helpful.

Stopping smoking is an important step in anyone's life. As you'll see, it isn't hard, but it requires some understanding by you of why you have continued to smoke.

You also need to be conscious of your lies to yourself about just having one and only one smoke, etc. You need to be wary of your own shtick, your song and dance to yourself of why you should have a cigarette. You need to be aware of the circumstances you need to avoid which result in that song and dance sounding convincing.

If it doesn't work the first time for you and you start smoking again, the way to deal with it is not to beat yourself up about it. Many people stop several times before they stop permanently. You learn something each time. *It's not a wasted effort.* You can't stop permanently before you can effectively deal with the stories you tell yourself to start smoking again.

The whole approach we're taking to stopping smoking is to get rid of your desire to smoke. But even if you do it successfully, that doesn't mean you will *never* have any desire to smoke. It does, however, mean that you will have 0 desire to smoke almost always. But you also have to deal with those few occasions when you *do* have some sort of desire to smoke.

The reason most people stop several times before they stop permanently is because they have to first acquire self-knowledge about the stories they tell themselves to start smoking again. They have to know how to avoid situations where those stories sound convincing (such as when you're drunk) and know how to handle those stories when we tell them to ourselves.

A famous such story is that you are going to just have one and only one cigarette. Another is that you need to smoke to deal with stress, or you need it to concentrate properly, or you need it to have a proper rest or break from work. One that I had to deal with several times was the lapse in judgment that occurs when I drink alcohol. I had to more or less stop drinking for several years to stop smoking.

The basic problem, when you're tempted to smoke, is that you want one. So the basic issue we need to address is how to get rid of that desire. Telling yourself you don't want it isn't going to stop you from wanting it.

The way to get rid of the desire to smoke is to dismantle the amplifier. The desire to smoke is actually a desire to alleviate stress, or calm fears, or a desire to focus and concentrate—or sometimes it's a desire for a break from work. Sometimes, such as when you've been drinking, it's a desire for 'enjoyment'.

Dismantling the amplifier, which is what this book is all about, is a matter of understanding at a very deep level that smoking doesn't give you any of those things. The amplifier is sustained by illusions that you will debunk. Once you disabuse yourself of the illusions that sustain the amplifier, your psychological dependence is on the way out.

You are a freedom fighter fighting for your own freedom from this addiction. The important thing is not to give up. Beating yourself up if you start again is not going to help you. Figuring out how you can do it better next time will, if you don't manage to stop permanently this time.

One of the things involved in stopping smoking permanently is giving yourself credit where credit is due for supplying yourself the things that you thought smoking was supplying. Smokers don't give themselves credit for that easily but they often think poorly of themselves for having tried and failed to stop smoking.

There are many novels where the hero looks like an idiot repeatedly but keeps trying. And eventually succeeds. We love that idiot. All of us are that idiot. Keep on trying. You are going to win.

It's a little bit like goaltending. Tending the goal. If the goalie lets in a goal, s/he can't get too upset about it because that will just cause her/him to let in more goals. They can't beat themselves up about it. Not even when it's a stinker of a goal. The worse the goal, the more important it is they don't beat themselves up about it and just get on with the job of making the next save. Just put it behind you and learn from it. Beating yourself up about it doesn't help anybody or anything. In fact it does you harm. It makes you think poorly of yourself, which can lead to bad decisions.

Smokers who start smoking again think that they didn't try hard enough or they lack will power or whatever. It's important to give yourself credit for being on the path to ditching this addiction once and for all. It takes a bit of practice for most people. But if you want it and keep at it, you *will* eventually triumph.

Hopefully what you learn the first time you read this book is exactly what you need to know to stop permanently this time. But even if it isn't permanent this time, you will have learned things that will eventually be crucial to your stopping smoking permanently.

Stopping permanently is a matter of getting to the point where you don't have illusions about smoking having any benefits to you whatsoever. Once you reach that point, you have dismantled the amplifier, you've dealt with the psychological addiction. The only reason you continue to smoke is this: you're convinced there's something in it for you. That and, of course, the physical addiction.

But the physical addiction is much easier to dispel than the brainwashing.

Getting rid of your illusions about smoking gets smoking out of your head. Getting it out of your heart is a related but slightly different thing. That's like getting an abusive lover out of your heart, or like getting the lust for cigarettes out of your system. It's easier to get an abuser out of your heart than to get Mr or Mrs Perfect out. Once you get smoking out of your head, the heart will not be far behind, though that may seem unlikely to you now.

If, when you finish this book, you think that you enjoy smoking, you have a serious illusion that is an impediment to successfully stopping smoking. The same goes for thinking that smoking provides you with stress relief, help with concentration, and help with relaxation. Similarly, if you think smoking tastes good at the end of this book — or provides you with anything good whatsoever — then you are likely to get back at it. Those illusions need to be dispelled.

If you start smoking again, look at it as one episode in a struggle you will eventually win. Once you have no illusions about smoking having any benefits, and the romance with smoking is over, you will not have any desire to smoke. But for some people that takes some time. For others, reading this book is just exactly what they need to permanently stop.

This book should change your outlook on smoking. You'll ditch smoking soon enough thereafter. Either by the end of the book or when your changed outlook catches up with you.

8 - Smoking and Illusions

Smoking is all about illusions. When we see someone smoking, we see their breath. We see the curl of imaginary things in the turbulence of its blue-gray path. Smoke is like a 'thought bubble' from comic books, only there are no words, just indistinct things in clouds of smoke. This is partly why smoking featured so frequently in movies, before it became dated rhetoric, dated practice. It offers a kind of smoky monologue without words in the acrid thought bubbles of tobacco smoke. It moves with the fluidity of air. A person's breathe and the way they're breathing is said to convey their spirit. Breathe is spirit. Smoking makes the spirit visible. It's all about illusions.

The visual illusions are not the only ones. What we think smoking gives us, it doesn't give us. That's all about illusions. The addiction is sustained only by illusions that you will dispel to free yourself from them.

Tobacco, of course, is not currently hallucinogenic. But the best studies of early tobacco usage (such as Johannes Wilbert's book *Tobacco and Shamanism in South America*) indicate that the shamans of some of the indigenous peoples of South America (tobacco came originally from South America) smoked strong enough versions of tobacco and smoked enough of it that it was indeed hallucinogenic—even while it first rendered them near-dead (sometimes truly dead) and catatonic. In any case, here again we see tobacco in relation to illusions—this time concerning literal hallucinations. Smoking involves illusions of various *types* including the hallucinatory tobacco usage of the "tobacco shamans".

Not only *people* but *states* are addicted to tobacco—and there's a big illusion which is central to the state's addiction to tobacco. States receive a great deal of revenue from tobacco sales, and have developed a strong dependence on it for hundreds of years. States think they get a lot of money from their addiction. But they're beginning to realize *that's an illusion*. It doesn't give them what they think it does. In fact, tobacco causes more strain on the state medical systems than it's worth. The medical bills from tobacco-related diseases outweigh the revenue from tobacco sales. Here we have a different type of tobacco addict—the state—but illusions are fundamental to the addiction. Dispelling that illusion is crucial to the state getting over its addiction.

Many of the indigenous peoples of the Americas prescribed tobacco medicinally for everything under the sun and used it in shamanic procedures extensively. Tobacco provides a strong illusion that it makes us feel better because of the relief it brings to nicotine withdrawal symptoms. It relieves the discomfort it itself causes via withdrawal symptoms. Here again we see tobacco in relation to illusion: it provides a good illusion that it helps with all sorts of medical conditions by providing relief from nicotine withdrawal symptoms. This is not a hallucination but a different type of illusion: an illusion of medicinal value.

Smoking was prescribed by doctors in the west for a variety of ailments even as late as the 1950's. It's no longer prescribed in the west at all, but it made its rounds in the medical establishment, providing the illusion of medicinal benefit for hundreds of years after its introduction to western society shortly after Europeans reached the Americas in 1492.

In a world where sometimes there is no easy cure for what ails us, an illusion can be comforting. Nicotine provides a convincing illusion that it makes us feel better by providing relief from the suffering of withdrawal symptoms it itself causes. It's like a con game in which the con artist says he's going to heal us. Instead, he poisons us. But the poison temporarily relieves the suffering the poison itself causes, later on. When he poisons us, he temporarily relieves our suffering (from the poison)—and guarantees more withdrawal symptoms in the future. Eventually the poison takes its toll on us and we struggle to escape the trap of the dependence it has established. But for a while—maybe decades, maybe until we die from it—the illusion the drug provides of feeling a bit better when we take it is important enough to us that we don't question it too much.

That's how it works now and that's probably how it worked about 5,000-9,000 years ago when people first started smoking tobacco in South America. It's very old, wanting badly enough to feel better that a poisonous, good illusion is better than nothing. The illusions associated with tobacco aren't now of the vivid hallucinogenic variety but are ones that we choose to believe, illusions that we believe to comfort ourselves. We choose to believe it's helping us and don't look very closely at the reality of the situation.

9 - The Addiction is Mainly Psychological

Reading a book can turn you into a non-smoker because the addiction depends on various illusions that a book can effectively debunk. Pills, gums, patches and other substances do not dismantle the psychological dependence. Addiction to nicotine is mostly psychological. By that I mean that the psychological addiction *amplifies* the physical desire for cigarettes. When smokers get 'cravings' for a cigarette, it's partly a desire for relief from nicotine withdrawal and it's partly a desire for the things you think smoking gives you such as concentration, relaxation, and relief from stress. If you understand the mechanics of your psychological addiction, you dismantle the amplifier. You dismantle the psychological addiction.

The actual physical addiction is *weak* without that amplifier. What you get without the amplifier at work are pathetic little twinges that don't have the power to make you do anything. And that's all that's left after you turn off the amplifier. The physical addiction lasts a few days after you've had your last cigarette. The physical sensation of withdrawal from nicotine is subtle, barely perceptible. If the amplifier is turned off, the sensation is like very mild hunger.

The notion that stopping smoking is necessarily an experience of deprivation and anxiety is a myth. A myth that serves to keep you in chains. It might as well be corporate propaganda straight from the tobacco companies, so widely believed and feared is it. It benefits the tobacco companies for you to believe it. You may say "It's no myth—I've tried to stop before and it was a difficult, exasperating experience that I don't want to repeat." I felt that way myself many times.

But there is a way to stop smoking that is enjoyable, empowering, educative about yourself, addiction, and the world, and it can be permanent in its cure. Even by the time you finish reading this book. It requires no special willpower. It just requires an open mind in reading the book and following the instructions. And a willingness to think about the reasons for why you continue to smoke.

You've already taken the first step. You're reading the book. Lots of people don't get this far. Sometimes because they're afraid that if they read it, they'll have to stop smoking. You don't have to stop if you don't want to. A book can't keep you from smoking. It can only show you how to stop if you want to. And, as I mentioned, you can smoke while you read the book as much as you please.

What you are going to do is dismantle the psychological addiction to smoking, the amplifier of the seemingly physical desire to smoke, by looking at it carefully and by understanding how it works. When you do that, when you understand the mechanisms, it's like understanding a magic trick. When you understand a magic trick, you are never ever fooled by it again.

Additionally, we will build a different amplifier: an amplifier of your joy, well-being and new found power and freedom from smoking. And that amplifier of joy and well-being will be powered by your understanding that you are indeed free from the slavery entailed in smoking. It will also be powered by your understanding of why you continued to smoke and your understanding that smoking does not, in fact, give you the things you thought it gave you. And you will be free to have everything that you thought smoking gave you—absolutely everything—and much more—but without smoking.

10 - You Will Never Enjoy Smoking Again

Life will be more enjoyable when you are finished reading this book. Not only can you be a non-smoker. You will also understand that the psychological addiction to cigarettes depends on brainwashing. Brainwashing that is partly instigated by tobacco companies but requires your own cooperation. You will learn how to stop cooperating in your own brainwashing about smoking and yourself.

You will never enjoy another cigarette after you read this book. Not because of scare tactics; I don't use scare tactics. Scare tactics don't work, for many people.

The reason why you won't enjoy another cigarette is because you will understand *you never really did enjoy them*. The idea that people enjoy smoking isn't accurate. They find *relief* in it from the withdrawal symptoms—they momentarily feel like a non-smoker. Smokers smoke to find relief from the withdrawal symptoms of nicotine addiction. Not because they enjoy smoking. Smokers smoke to temporarily feel like a non-smoker. Smokers smoke because they are addicted to nicotine.

Many smokers recognize that they don't enjoy smoking. It makes their heart pound. It tastes like an ashtray. It makes them smelly. It covers the area in nicotine. The ashes get all over things. It devalues your home. Smokers are not welcome in most places. It makes them wheeze and cough. It makes them sick and anxious. They are less physically active than non-smokers. It costs a lot of money. The money goes to people who make a product that kills millions of people. Smokers experience the existential dread of knowing that it could kill them eventually.

But smokers feel trapped by the need to find relief from the withdrawal symptoms. They tell themselves they enjoy smoking and so lose a sense of what real enjoyment is.

Enjoyment shouldn't be confused with temporary relief from irritation. Just like we wouldn't confuse enjoyment with the relief people feel when they stop banging their head against a wall. Similarly, we wouldn't confuse enjoyment with the feeling you'd get paying someone to temporarily go away—someone who won't leave you alone unless you pay them to go away for thirty minutes.

11 - This Book Does Not Use Scare Tactics

We won't be using scare tactics any more than dispelling illusions about card tricks requires scare tactics. *To dispel illusions about card tricks, you don't need to scare anybody. You just look at what is really going on and how that creates an illusion.* You just show people what is really going on. Once you understand that *you have never truly enjoyed cigarettes* and understand why you think you do enjoy them, and understand they don't give you what you thought they did, you will never be under the illusion again that you enjoy a cigarette.

12 - Dumbo and the Feather

One of my main impediments to stopping smoking was the feeling that it helped me with the ability to concentrate. As a writer, I need that badly. I was convinced that I just wouldn't be as good without being able to smoke.

As it turns out, of course, I wasn't giving myself enough credit. It turns out that I can concentrate better without smoking. Smoking creates distracting withdrawal symptoms. Without those, it's possible to concentrate for longer periods.

My situation was a bit like that of Dumbo the elephant, the main character from the 1941 Disney movie of the same name. Dumbo had huge ears that allowed him to fly. But Dumbo didn't believe he could fly until the crows gave him a feather. When Dumbo had the feather with him, he found he could fly. He thought he couldn't fly without it. Coming to the realization that he didn't need the feather to fly was an important part of the movie. And of Dumbo's growth.

No writer ever got up and thanked her cigarettes for help with that prize-winning novel. Turns out it was me, all along, helping me to concentrate. The cigarettes were just a ' feather' that I didn't need.

All those years I smoked, I thought it was helping me concentrate. It would be easy to beat myself up about it. But, you know, Dumbo might never have flown if the crows hadn't given him the feather. Dumbo apparently needed the feather to *start* flying.

And then he needed to realize he didn't need it to fly.

Similarly, there were probably times when smoking helped you to 'fly' because you didn't think you could do it without it. You found you could, with the help of the ' cigarette'. But now it's time to see you don't need it and it isn't giving you anything anymore. On the contrary, it's keeping you down, now.

13 - The Illusion of Enjoying Cigarettes

Nicotine provides a strong illusion of enjoyment. Smokers feel the discomfort of withdrawal symptoms. Taking the drug temporarily releases them from the discomfort of withdrawal symptoms. This is what eventually passes for enjoyment. Addictive drugs provide both suffering and relief from the suffering.

To mistake *relief* from withdrawal symptoms for *enjoyment* is like thanking the con man who's robbing you blind for the gifts he gives you to keep you from looking too carefully at what he's doing to you.

The idea that addicts enjoy the drug debases the meaning of *enjoyment*. Enjoyment involves experiencing something more than the removal of suffering which the drug itself caused. When we eat a good meal, we experience the nutritional benefit of the food and the tastiness, and sometimes the social pleasure of eating with others. We need food, and good food nourishes us. So it makes sense to say we enjoyed a good meal, but to say we enjoyed a cigarette is to be under several illusions that keep you smoking. How can you enjoy something that simply dispels the incessant irritation that it itself causes? One is so grateful for relief from irritation that we think we enjoy what provides the pain and the relief from the pain.

Smokers tell themselves they enjoy smoking and that it helps them concentrate. But it only provides the illusion of helping with concentration by temporarily removing its withdrawal symptoms. Just as it provides the illusion of relaxation by temporarily removing withdrawal symptoms. Smokers are under the illusion that they need to smoke to feel right. To feel good. To enjoy life. Because they think smoking gives them things that smoking doesn't give them at all.

Once you understand that smoking doesn't give you any of the good things/feelings you thought it was giving you, an apparently miraculous thing happens: the urges disappear. You're going to experience it and then you're going to see that it's no miracle. Tobacco addictions depend on smoky illusions that dissipate and dissolve in the light of understanding. But my own illusions about smoking kept me at it for thirty years. They can be very powerful while you are under their spell. However, they are also easy to remove if you know how. And that's exactly what we're going to do.

14 - Getting Rid of the 'Urge' to Smoke

Once you understand why you continued to smoke and also understand that smoking doesn't give you what you thought it was giving you, the psychological amplifier of desire for cigarettes is dealt an irreparable blow: you know you don't need to smoke. You don't need it to get the *genuinely important* things you *thought* it was giving you. Because you know smoking isn't giving you those things at all.

Once you know that, then the urge to smoke 'mysteriously'—almost miraculously—disappears. Let's remove the mystery.

It disappears because 99% of the urge to smoke is *psychological*. The psychological portion of the urge is not an urge to smoke but is an urge for what you think smoking gives you, whether that is concentration, relaxation, enjoyment, stress management, or whatever. When you understand that it's not actually giving you any of those important things, you understand you don't need to smoke to get any of them. And then you don't amplify desire for those important things into strong urges to smoke cigarettes.

Figure out the things you thought you were getting from smoking. Different people think it gives them different things. There are typical ones such as concentration, relaxation, stress management, weight management and so on. But it can also be about belonging to a group. Or making a connection with a parent if your parents smoked. Many people started smoking to appear to be adults; they were kids wanting to be adults.

Whatever the reasons were that you *started*, the reasons why you *continue* to smoke more recently are the really important ones now. Because they tell you what you think smoking is giving you now. You *must* think smoking is giving you important things/feelings for you to continue. Important enough that you're willing to put up with a lot of poison to get those things, you think, from smoking. You need to reflect on what you think you're getting from smoking. Once you figure that out, you are a lot closer to the goal.

It's easy to show you that smoking doesn't give you what you thought you were getting from it. The hard part is figuring out what you think it's giving you. Understanding that it doesn't give you those things at all is straightforward, for the most part; *you supply them yourself* and could supply them yourself even better without smoking.

There are doctors, such as Vancouver's Gabor Maté, who say that all addictions, whether to nicotine, heroin, sex—or whatever—are basically attempts to self-medicate traumas that typically were suffered in childhood. The idea is that early trauma creates an ongoing state of anxious insecurity that we sometimes seek to assuage through addictions of one sort or another. The object of the addiction (the drug or whatever) is self-medication to alleviate the fear/insecurity/pain/trauma that has created a situation where we feel we are in need of something to make us feel better.

An addiction is consumption that the addict feels compelled to persist in even even when they want to stop and when they experience negative consequences for not stopping. This definition of addiction does not require a drug that is physically addictive. It emphasizes the psychological dimension of addiction as the dominant aspect. In untethering the notion of addiction from necessarily involving dependence on a substance, the focus shifts to psychological dependency. To say it's mostly in the head doesn't make it an easier problem, but it clarifies what's really going on.

Psychological addiction involves the idea that you need the thing consumed very badly in an ongoing manner. You need it to get something important you can't have without it—or so you think. Determining what those things are is sometimes available to you fairly easily by introspection. For other people, it's more difficult to determine what those things are because they are lost in the mists of anxiety and insecurity that goes back to childhood. Or for some other reason you're keeping secrets from yourself.

Be that as it may, you *may* not actually need to understand your psychological issues at that deep level in order to cure yourself of addiction to smoking. Here's why. You need to understand and accept and embrace the truth that smoking does not give you the important things that you thought it gave you. Whether you understand those important things to be the typical things—concentration, relaxation, stress reduction, and so on—or the assuaging of your deepest insecurities about your ability to cope on your own without a 'crutch' like a cigarette—in either case, you need to understand and accept that smoking does not give you *anything at all* that is important to you.

That means your *head* is in the right place. But you also need to have a change of *heart* about smoking. You need to end the romance. Just like with a personal relationship, you need to think about it both in terms of your head and your heart. Urges to smoke are desires to smoke. Desire to smoke is amplified by the romance just as it is by the need for concentration or relaxation or whatever.

15 - The Romance

Let me clarify what I mean by 'the romance with smoking'.

People look for a kind of escape in smoking. A smoke-break is a break from or escape from work. It's like a little holiday. Well, that's a kind of a romantic view of a smoke-break, isn't it. It's like a little trip to Paris. No, it's not, but we romanticize smoking as an escape. It's a little intoxication to relax in preparation for labor. Or at least it's some relief from the distraction it itself causes via withdrawal symptoms.

The romance with smoking has many aspects just like a romance between people has many aspects. We like a romance with another person to take us away from our troubles, to provide relaxation, enjoyment, and emotional solace.

Some people think of their cigarette as their "little friend who is always there for me". It isn't simply that they associate cigarettes with the ability to concentrate and relax. They have an emotional attachment to cigarettes.

But the romance can also be about thinking smoking is cool or otherwise attractive. 'Romance' doesn't necessarily apply solely to a relationship between two people. It involves emotional attachment and being 'romanced', seduced, swept away; it involves fantasies of the object of the romance providing all manner of good things and perhaps living happily ever after.

The history of tobacco smoking overflows with ideas of smoking as a panacea, a cure-all, a boon to humanity. A god, even, or the food of the gods. Many of the indigenous peoples of the Americas believed that offering the spirits tobacco was an offer spirits literally could not refuse; the spirits would grant the supplicant's wish in return for the tobacco which the spirits craved intensely. Here we see tobacco as something you had to have to get your needs fulfilled, to have your prayers answered. That is beyond a romance with tobacco; that is religious use of tobacco. Even the spirits craved and needed it.

More typically, there is the romance of escape from drudgery, boring work. A smoke break is a brief escape into the romance of nicotine-induced relaxation. The meaning of the Marlboro Man is that it's an image of freedom from the drudgery of civilization.

It's ironic that while we romanticize smoking into something that offers escape from, freedom from troubles, worry, work and whatnot, it's an addiction that exacts a certain servitude. The romance with smoking is abusive, in the end. It takes but gives nothing, really.

Self-knowledge is important to moving forward in life, and so it is in the case of stopping smoking. The things you think smoking gives you must be very important to you: you've been willing to poison yourself to the point of illness to get them. The point is that people usually think smoking helps them deal with their deepest issues. You need to ask yourself what those are, and whether you use smoking to deal with them.

If so, then I have some very good news for you. All this time that you've been smoking, smoking hasn't helped you one little bit with those deep issues; *you've managed on your own*, a task that would be easier without the illusion that smoking was any help at all. It's like you've had this freeloader on board who takes credit for helping you but, in reality, is no help at all and, in fact, poisons you and adds more stress to your life rather than reducing it.

Dismantling your psychological addiction *permanently* involves having a grasp on why you continued to smoke, ie, an understanding of the *full range* of what you thought smoking was providing you, and a strong understanding of why it does not provide those things at all.

When you get there, you'll know it. The prospect of starting to smoke again will be as improbable to you as the prospect of being fooled by a card trick that you understand. All the old con jobs you tell yourself to have a cigarette will sound exactly like con jobs promising things that smoking doesn't deliver. You won't want a cigarette, and you will know you can't be made to want one by other people. And it will be harder for you to fool yourself on the matter. Nobody fools us better than we ourselves do.

16 - How Long Until You're Hooked?

Is it the first cigarette? The tenth? The twentieth? When are you hooked? You're hooked when you want one. You're hooked when you think you'll enjoy it, that cigarettes are enjoyable. You're hooked when you believe the proffered illusions: that it has something to offer you that you need, that it helps you relax, concentrate, that it gives you maturity in the eyes of your peers, or toughness, rebelliousness, a bond with other addicts, or any of the other illusions. You're hooked when you believe it's going to help you in any way whatsoever, when you're seduced by the romance of smoking.

You're hooked like a fish when you want to smoke. You're simply landed when you smoke it. You're hooked before you smoke your first cigarette. You're landed when you smoke it. And, after you're landed, you're thrown back in—with the hook in your mouth via the physical addiction.

People who stop smoking for years but still believe some of the illusions about smoking go back to it because they are still hooked, even though they are no longer physically addicted. Those illusions are crucial to the addiction. Those who see these illusions for what they are—illusions—rarely go back. It's like understanding how a 'magic' trick works. Once you do, the 'magic' of that trick is permanently dispelled.

The linch pin of addiction is desire for the object of the addiction. If you want it, you're hooked, even if you're not consuming it. And how do you get over desire for it? You realize it isn't providing you with what you thought it was providing you. Nothing and nobody can, except you, provide you with that. You already provide yourself what you thought it was providing you. It doesn't give you that at all. You don't give yourself enough credit. And once you realize that the object of the addiction does not give you the very important things you thought it was providing you, a seemingly magical thing happens. You don't want it anymore.

But it isn't magical. It's just that the urges for the object of the addiction are really your amplified desires for what you thought the object was providing you. Yes you really need those things but the object of the addiction isn't giving you those things at all. You give them to yourself. You always did. It never did. And once you realize that, the illusion is over. And you don't want it anymore. And you are free of it.

Dismantling the psychological addiction to smoking is something you look at from the head and the heart. What is your emotional connection to smoking? What is the nature of the romance with smoking, for you?

That romance has an irrational dimension to it. People can intellectually know that a lover is abusive, that they shouldn't stay, that the lover doesn't love them, that the lover does not meet their needs and is only a parasite. Yet they sometimes stay because they love him/her. They feel they can't live without her/him.

The romance is still alive, for them. The attraction still exists. Sometimes it's because although they know that the lover is an abusive parasite which, make no mistake, is what smoking is, they don't feel that they themselves deserve to be free of the parasite. In such case, they have to give themselves some credit, credit that is due to them. *Nobody deserves to be somebody's punching bag or to be emotionally abused. And nobody deserves to be enslaved to an addiction that robs them of health, money, and self-respect.*

If you took up smoking long ago to be a rebel, now is the time to truly rebel against the slavery of addiction. To stop smoking, to end the romance, you need to assert your self-worth in the face of this abusive addiction. You don't need smoking. Everything you thought it gave you, it doesn't. Everything you thought it gave you, you've been giving yourself, all this time. It's a vampire sucking on your blood. It's a parasite. It doesn't care if you live or die. End that romance.

17 - "Giving up" vs "Quitting" vs "Stopping" Smoking

To 'quit' or to 'give up' smoking is different from 'stopping' smoking. Usually, people who say they 'quit smoking' or they 'want to quit smoking' feel that they did or would be giving up something of great importance to them. The implication usually is that 'quitting smoking' involves a sacrifice and hardship.

If the implication of sacrifice is only occasional and slight when people say they "quit smoking", it's much stronger and direct when they say they "gave up smoking".

The way you're going about it, though, is different. You are going to 'stop smoking'. There is no sacrifice or hardship involved. You get everything you had when smoking, only better. And you get many things you didn't have when you smoked, such as better health, less stress, better relaxation, better concentration, more money in your pocket, and no servitude to the Mordor corporation.

I had a surprising conversation with a dear friend who has not smoked for 17 years and who was the one who alerted me about the existence of Allen Carr's book several years ago.

She said "I gave up 17 years ago (tobacco) and still think about it."

This surprised me and I replied "You mean you still want it?"

She said "Yes, not all the time - just when in 'thinking hard' mode... it helped, darn it."

The poor woman is still hooked. You're hooked when you want it. You're landed when you smoke it. If you think there's something for you in it, you want it. She thinks it helped her with concentration. She "gave up" smoking, but it still has a little grip on her. At important moments in her life. 'Thinking hard' mode is important to her as it is to me.

Smoking only 'helps' with concentration and creativity by removing withdrawal symptoms it itself causes. One is temporarily free, when one smokes, from withdrawal symptoms. One is temporarily free from desire. One is suddenly blank. One is suddenly open. For creative and/or intellectual people, that is an important state because creation rushes into that fresh void.

Smoking allows smokers to get there: to blankness, to relief from desire. But it isn't something that smokers absolutely require to get there. They think it is because it's pretty tough for smokers to get there with withdrawal symptoms getting in the way.

But creative people get there without smoking. My friend does. Her work is marvelous. Especially these days. Think of the blankness. Think of how it feels to be free from desire. Think of how it feels to be blank. Be blank. There. You have it. Without smoking.

18 - The End of the Romance

Getting rid of an addiction is not exactly the same as getting rid of an exploitative, abusive lover, but they are not unrelated.

Smokers imagine the relation with their cigarettes in all sorts of ways from that of a loyal friend to, yes, a lover, to the pill that makes everything better, to an indispensable ally who helps deal with stress, helps us celebrate, helps us relax, and so on.

Many will describe their having stopped smoking as a falling out of love with smoking. And perhaps as a falling in love with a new day of freedom for them.

People addicted to cigarettes sometimes cannot imagine life being worth living without cigarettes in their life, like a mate to whom one is profoundly attached.

Cigarettes aren't your friend, ally, and cigarettes do not contribute to your well-being. Instead, they harm you very seriously in several ways. If smoking is like a romance, it's like an *abusive* relationship.

If you have successfully and permanently ended relationships where you were in love but came to see that the relationship had to end, you can bring that experience to this situation to help you fall out of love with smoking. You know how it's done. And this abuser *really deserves the boot*.

Additionally, if you come to realize how much more enjoyable life is without that murderous vampire sucking the life out of you, you can truly begin to love life without smoking.

To 'end the romance' with smoking is to no longer desire to smoke. To get to the point where you no longer desire to smoke cigarettes is to have ended the romance.

To stay that way, you need to be clear about how smoking did not give you the things you thought you were getting from smoking, and that you can even better obtain those things without smoking.

Also, to stay clear, cultivate your joy and happiness at being a non-smoker. You need to be able to feel that and appreciate that joy, happiness, and freedom when smoking propositions you, as will happen occasionally .

So let's try it right now. Can you feel the joy of freedom from smoking? It's a relief the intensity of which dwarfs the relief you experienced when smoking a cigarette. Your future looks different and inviting; it's a relief that you will soon be feeling so much better, that you are more in charge of your own life. In addition to being a relief, there's a sense of strength and anticipation about moving forward in life. There's anticipation and curiosity about feeling better. And anticipation about taking your new body out for a spin. Exercise feels great when you stop smoking. And there's amazement and wonder in this experience. You see more clearly. You are no longer fooling yourself about smoking helping you, or being necessary in your life. There are other benefits to stopping smoking we will touch on. Count your blessings, feel the joy, rejoice in your freedom, and appreciate the weakness of the little monster's dying twitches.

Take a deep breath. Feel the pleasure in breathing deeply. Your lung capacity increases over time after you stop smoking. We'll talk more about appreciating the pleasure of breathing deeply, appreciating the pleasure of breathing and feeling infused with energy when you breath fresh air. You'll be surprised to learn that this experience was actually important to George Lucas's inspiration for 'the force' in Star Wars. When you breath deeply, you do indeed experience 'the force', which is *prana*, or the life force. You are infused with it when you breath fresh air deeply. But more about that later.

Enjoy the knowledge that you will never pay the vampire tobacco companies another penny. You won't be paying your own assassins. You are no longer financing your own slow execution. You are no longer paying money to tobacco companies that sell people poison. You aren't giving them money to create and sell a product that is a poisonous confidence game. You are no longer buying the toxic, disgusting lies they sell to so many people: that cigarettes are enjoyable, relaxing, stress reducing, good for concentration, etc.

If you have dismantled the amplifier of desire for cigarettes, you can see it in front of you like a disassembled robot, the springs, sprockets and widgets of which are lying all over the floor, never to come together again into the instrument of oppression and brainwashing that it was for so long. You understand how that machine works now. You understand the trick of enslavement to smoking. It won't work on you again if you retain your current understanding and deepen it over time.

19 - Sex and Smoking

The urge to smoke has different facets. One facet is desire for relief from withdrawal symptoms, desire to dispel the mild hunger that withdrawal symptoms entail.

Another facet is the desire to allay fears, anxieties, and insecurities of daily life. Our fears and anxieties often bother us more than withdrawal symptoms from nicotine do. They amplify the withdrawal symptoms which, on their own, are merely twinges of something like mild hunger. The urge to have a cigarette is not simply caused by the physical symptoms of nicotine addiction. It's charged, amplified with the psychic energy of our fears, anxieties and insecurities which we desire to allay in the act of smoking.

The urge to smoke can also be associated with relief from work. The smoke-break is a short escape into the romance of smoking.

Another facet of the urge can be sexual. The urge to smoke, for some people, is sometimes lusty, a desire for the pounding heart and release of sexual energy in the way the smoke can sometimes render one limp and dizzy. The urge for a cigarette sometimes is feral, fierce, amplified by sexuality.

There can be an element of intoxication. The arc of stimulation followed by relaxation in the experience of smoking is similar to the arc of sex where first there is stimulation followed by relief and relaxation.

All of these aspects can be thought of as part of the romance with smoking. Romance isn't simply a matter of sex but of reliance concerning many other needs. But the sort of urgency associated with one's sex drive can sometimes be quite similar to the urge to smoke, so that libidinous urges are a part of the romance with smoking.

There was undeniably an element of sexuality in my own addiction. When I quit smoking several times before I read Allen Carr's book, I would eventually experience a kind of lust very like I was *stalking* a cigarette—though I assure you I am not a stalker of *people*. Maybe not today, maybe not tomorrow, but it was a foregone conclusion that eventually I would satisfy my lust for a cigarette.

Both my parents were smokers. I started smoking stealing my

mother's cigarettes at the age of twelve. I smoked my first cigarette in puberty when I wanted to be an adult. Smoking was one of what seemed like very few adult avenues that I could sneak into.

That there is a sexual dimension to smoking is recognized but not widely discussed. For years, in cinema, smoking symbolized smoldering passion, lusty desire. When you light someone else's cigarette, it ignites other associations. There is an aging stereotype of couples smoking in bed after sex. And so on. The image of the hot rebellious youth smoking is much beloved by cigarette companies.

These days, you don't see smoking in Hollywood films or on TV as much as in the past. However, the Internet is the new playground for tobacco advertising; it isn't regulated like so many other media spheres have been. Porn sites have vast libraries of naked people smoking while they have sex.

The sexual, for some—probably for most and perhaps all—is a prominent part of their psychological addiction.

How do you ditch that? How do you end the romance in your heart —and groin—with smoking? Being clear in the head helps considerably, like it does in interpersonal relationships. Being clear that it isn't giving you what you thought it was giving you. And that it is, instead, all take take take. It takes your health, your money, your self-respect, on and on. After you've killed the *little monster*, after you haven't smoked for a week, smoking doesn't even provide relief from withdrawal symptoms. It just knocks you down.

If there's a romance involved in smoking, it's an abusive relationship. You just gotta have it, and it gives you abuse in return. It even impairs your sexuality, in the long run. Smoking is bad for your circulation. Nicotine constricts blood vessels, and for your sexual organs to work optimally, good circulation is required—in both males and females.

My own romance with smoking was something I wondered if I could *ever* change. It felt like trying to change my sexual preference. But it isn't that way. It might not be instantaneous, but you will find that eventually the romance is truly over in your heart. It's more like getting a bad relationship out of your heart than changing your sexual preference.

Getting over a bad romance emotionally can sometimes take longer than getting clear in your head that it's definitely for the best it's at an end. But if you're clear about it in your head, the heart catches up with you before long.

The heart shouldn't be too far behind the head in this case because it's so dramatically an *abusive* relationship. Smoking abuses your body and your mind. The health effects are well-known. It's a serial killer beyond the scope of Hitler or Stalin. It also is bad for your sexual performance, not only because nicotine constricts arteries, but because it damages so many organs, including the lungs, which quickly leaves you out of breath and wheezing.

But the abuse is also mental. You think you need and want something that, to you, looks lovely and desirable but, in fact, looks like the ugliest of blood-suckers sucking on your neck. The romance is one-way. You like it but it doesn't like you one bit. It will kill you eventually and toss you away like a cigarette butt.

That's harsh, but six million people perish of smoking-related diseases every year; that's expected to rise to eight million by 2030.

Getting to the point where the romance with smoking is over, for you, can happen as it sometimes happens in personal relationships where you can remember the precise moment you were over it.

That is the moment when the veil of illusion is lifted. That is the moment when you see that smoking doesn't give you what you thought it was giving you. You have this experience one by one concerning all your illusions about what smoking gives you.

One of those illusions can be that smoking is delicious like sex is delicious. One's desire to smoke is experienced like one's desire for sex, and smoking is experienced like the transport of sex.

But, eventually, your image of this is less of *Eros* and more of *Thanatos*. What does that mean? *Eros* is the figure of love. *Thanatos* is the figure of death. You had previously thought of and, perhaps more importantly, *felt* the desire to smoke as the desire for life, for enjoyment, for relaxation, for the relief of stress, for concentration, for inspiration and so on. And you'd felt smoking to be pleasurable, even as pleasurable as sex.

But, eventually, when you think about smoking, you don't feel something like sexual desire. The thought of the drug entering your system feels like poison entering your bloodstream. And you experience gentleness and pity for yourself that you previously identified that feeling with the good things in life.

Be gentle with yourself. Don't reprove yourself about it. Don't blame yourself for it. Blaming yourself is just more personal abuse. Getting free of it is the important thing.

You feel that you do not want to be poisoned. You feel it as a kind of chemical violence to your body that is not pleasureful but violently abusive. That's eventually how you feel about it.

Then you take a deep breath of fresh air. As we will see later in the book, cultivating an appreciation for that pleasure, the simple pleasure of breathing fresh air, is an appreciation of life, not of death.

20 - Tobacco Companies Are Counting On You

The first draft of this chapter was much angrier at tobacco companies. It was about how tobacco companies count on you to be a reliable addict and how you pay them for poison for a long but prematurely early time. It was very angry. But how should we feel about tobacco companies?

Tobacco has been sold in various forms in the west for about 500 years, since it was brought to Europe from the Americas. It's really only since the 1950's, though, that medical research into the effects of smoking has proved beyond *any* doubt that smoking is addictive and extraordinarily bad for your health. Prior to that time, tobacco companies could pretend ignorance about the damage they do. But now they cannot. Their perfidy is plainly visible to all who care to see. They sell a product that kills millions of people each year.

> Tobacco use is the leading preventable cause of death in the United States.[1]

These are the sort of companies you definitely would prefer not to support. Contributing to their revenue is like supporting the Mordor Corporation.

It used to be that smoking and smokers were seen as cool, fashionable, elegant, and sexy. Tobacco company advertising made it so. In the 1950's, artists, intellectuals, beatniks, rebels and free-thinkers of all stripes smoked. But the social meaning of smoking has undergone a *total and complete reversal* in the west from the 1950's.

Now, rather than being associated with freedom—of any description—it's associated with addiction, dependence, slavery—with the opposite of freedom. And rather than being associated with health and vitality, it's associated with illness, dissolution and death. Rather than being associated with the rebel, it's associated with slavish corporate consumerism. That is how the ideology of smoking is perceived now. That is now the predominant social meaning of smoking.

---

1 From cdc.gov/tobacco/data_statistics/fact_sheets/health_effects/tobacco_rel ated_mortality

The 'benefits' of smoking have been shown to be illusions, and the drawbacks have been proved to be profound both on individuals and on society as a whole. The strain on the medical system caused by smoking-related diseases is significant. The state pays more for the health-care of smokers than it reaps in revenue from smokers buying cigarettes. The state has enough information to get over its addiction to revenue from tobacco.

The response of tobacco companies to all this has always been resistance and denial, as far as possible. And when that failed, they sought to capitalize on foreign markets where regulation was not as strong. Smoking rates in developing countries are much higher than in the west; tobacco companies are making hay while the sun shines there.

> Smoking in Indonesia is common, as there are approximately 57 million smokers in Indonesia. Of Indonesian people, 63% of men and 5% of women reported being smokers, a total of 34% of the population.[2]

As smoking rates continue to decrease in the west, tobacco companies will turn to alternative nicotine addictions such as 'electronic cigarettes' for revenue and will claim that they are harmless as long as they possibly can, until the research catches up with them again.

'Electronic cigarettes' are probably not as toxic as regular cigarettes. But do not expect good things from merchants of death, even though tobacco companies are counting on you.

How do tobacco companies count on you? They count on you like one counts on a statistic. That's what you are to them: an anonymous statistic. They will not, of course, be very big on contact with their customers.

It's important to understand the perspective on you that tobacco companies count on. They're counting on you to be frightened of the truth. They're counting on your insecurities defeating you. They're betting against you. But you deserve to kick their butt, and you will.

They know that smoking doesn't give you anything good or valuable.

---

2   From en.wikipedia.org/wiki/Smoking_in_Indonesia .

They know it doesn't really help you concentrate or be relaxed. They know all that very well indeed. This con game business has been much the same for 500 years in the west. Help the customer think they need the product, that it's indispensable to them. This is not unique to the cigarette business. That's how many things are advertised and sold.

They know that the only things keeping you smoking are illusions about what you get from smoking. So what could their strategy be to keep you smoking? Their strategy has been, continues to be, and will always be to bet on your weaknesses. If they bet on your strengths, they'd be betting on losing you as a customer. So they bet on your weaknesses because cigarettes play on your weaknesses. Their product is so terrible that's all they can do. They've got a terrible product for you—so terrible that the only thing that can help them keep you coming back is appealing to your weaknesses and your fear.

They want you to think that you have weaknesses that make you *need* to smoke. They want you to think that you can't concentrate very well on your own. They want you to think you need to smoke to concentrate well. They want you to fear the prospect of not smoking just exactly like you fear the prospect of not being able to have the important things you think smoking gives you.

They're counting on you not being able to enjoy life without cigarettes. They want you to think that your confidence and enjoyment of life, your ability to handle stress, your relaxation, your very well-being depends on your ability to smoke. The stronger your illusion that you need their poison to function happily and effectively, the better they like it.

As long as your fears and insecurities are strong enough to make you think you actually need the revolting poisons they peddle to 'enjoy' life, they know you're a dependable consumer. What they don't want you to realize is that you don't need their product at all.

They want you to fear stopping smoking. But I'm telling you it's one of the best experiences you can have. You're going to see and understand that stopping smoking permanently is largely a matter of making a big change in your perspective on smoking.

21 - Changing your Perspective

A change in perspective can change a lot of things. There's a sculpture of Nelson Mandela by Marco Cianfanelli on the site of Mandela's capture by the South African authorities that led to his imprisonment for 27 years. The sculpture is composed of 50 steel columns which, when viewed from one perspective, form an image of Mandela's face. When viewed from other perspectives, the 50 steel columns give no hint of resembling a face. The sculpture reminds us, among other things, that *what we see depends on our perspective.*

Sometimes our perspective presents us with a perfect illusion that seems solid, undeniable, and as real as the nose on your face—or on Mandela's face. Yet if we shift our perspective, the situation can look very different. The nose and face disappear altogether. The illusion disappears. *And you never ever think of it again as you did before.*

We're going to examine the perspectives smokers have on the typical reasons why they continue to smoke. We're going to look at alternative perspectives. The alternative perspectives reveal the illusory nature of smokers' attitudes to what smoking gives them. Smokers believe smoking gives them genuinely important things in their life, things that non-smokers value highly also. Things that we need to enjoy life. And smokers believe they can't have those things without smoking.

We're going to look at what those things typically are. We're going to examine alternative perspectives on whether smoking provides them. Smoking doesn't provide any of the benefits that are associated with it. You provide those things to yourself by yourself and always have. The world is full of myths about the benefits of smoking. Myths that are easily debunked if you keep an open mind.

Once those myths are debunked, you realize you don't need to smoke, you realize it isn't giving you anything of value, you realize that all it's giving you is trouble, and the urge to smoke disappears.

Your perspective was fixed to one point of view that presented a perfect illusion about the benefits of smoking. But you develop new perspectives so you can walk around and see the matter from different points of view, like walking around the Mandela sculpture and seeing it from different angles.

22 - Twentieth Century Artists and Smoking

I've seen many pictures of 20th century writers smoking. It used to be almost a job requirement, it seems, for writers to smoke. That and heavy drinking. It gives you pause to consider how well-fooled they were. Many of them died from smoking. The best writers in the world. Some of the most intelligent, creative people in the world. These writers who were all about chasing down the truth of things.

If they couldn't see through the lies and illusions, why can we?

You can do it because *those writers didn't understand what they were dealing with but you do.* They didn't understand what they were dealing with concerning health issues. But understanding the health issues is not very helpful when you're trying to stop. We all now know how toxic smoking is, but it doesn't help us stop as much as you'd hope. Why? Because it does nothing to diminish the desire for a cigarette. Fear does not diminish our desire for cigarettes. What gets rid of our desire to smoke is understanding what good things we think it's giving us and understanding it doesn't actually give us those things at all.

The artists of the 20th century didn't understand what they were dealing with—and, also, they didn't understand how to deal with it.

Those writers lived in a time when even the king of England smoked heavily and died of it. King George VI died at age 57 in 1952. He was prescribed smoking by his doctors for his speech impediment. He was one of the great leaders Britain had during World War II. The Nazis didn't get him—he played an important role in their defeat—but smoking did.

People did not understand that smoking has no benefits. But you are coming to that understanding in a serious way.

Back in the 1950's doctors prescribed smoking for things such as weight loss and stress management. When doctors prescribe something, people tend to think of it as indeed being medicinal. It was as though there was a terrible villain masquerading as everyone's friend and helper. It even managed to kill the King before it was unmasked.

Now we know what we're dealing with. And how to deal with it.

23 - The Number of Smokers World-Wide

Decades of solid, undisputed medical research in the west link cigarette smoking to assorted types of cancer, strokes, coronary heart disease, and many other diseases.

> Cigarette smoking causes more than 480,000 deaths each year in the United States. This is about one in five deaths.[3]

Laws banning cigarette advertising and smoking in public places have been widely implemented. Laws making it illegal to sell tobacco products to minors are common. However, although smoking rates have been dropping for the last quarter century in western countries, in Canada in 2012, 16% of the adult population smoked. Similar rates held in the USA:

> Cigarette smoking has decreased among adults in the United States from about 42% of the population in 1965 to about 18% in 2012 (the latest year for which numbers are available). But it's still the most common form of tobacco use in the US: about 42 million (somewhat fewer than 1 in every 5) adults currently smoke cigarettes.[4]

Much the same story is told in England:

> In Britain in 1948, when surveys of smoking began, smoking was extremely prevalent among men: 82% smoked some form of tobacco and 65% were cigarette smokers. By 1970, the percentage of male cigarette smokers had fallen to 55%. From the 1970s onward, smoking prevalence fell rapidly until the mid-1990s. Since then the rate has continued to fall slowly and in 2007 around a fifth (22%) of men (aged 16 and over)

---

3   From
    cdc.gov/tobacco/data_statistics/fact_sheets/health_effects/effects_cig_
    smoking (2015)

4   From
    cancer.org/cancer/cancercauses/tobaccocancer/questionsaboutsmokin
    gtobaccoandhealth/ questions-about-smoking-tobacco-and-health-
    how-many-use (2015)

were reported as cigarette smokers. Between 2007 and 2009, the rate remained stable, and fell to 21% in 2010.[5]

The current numbers in Australia are much the same[6]. In Germany, the rates are higher:

> According to a 2013 micro-census survey, 24.5% of the German population aged 15+ are smokers (29 percent in men, 20 percent in women). Among the 18- to 25-year-old age group, 35.2% are smokers.[7]

In many parts of the world, little or no legislation is in place to prevent tobacco companies from killing millions of people. China has the most smokers in the world. In 2015 about half the male adult population were smokers. Less than 5% of the adult female population smokes. Smoking kills about *1.2 million Chinese people annually.*

> ...China is the world's largest consumer and producer of tobacco: there are 350 million Chinese smokers, and China produces 42% of the world's cigarettes. The China National Tobacco Corporation is by sales the largest single manufacturer of tobacco products in the world and boasts a monopoly in Mainland China generating between 7% to 10% of government revenue....Tobacco is still a ubiquitous gift acceptable on any occasion, particularly outside of urban areas....Smoking is considered socially acceptable anywhere at any time, even if it is technically illegal.

> ...progress on tobacco control is not moving quickly because the government derives large tax revenues from tobacco sales, and the industry employs a large workforce....A study conducted among 800 Chinese male surgeons in 2004 found that 45.2% were

5   From cancerresearchuk.org/about-cancer/causes-of-cancer/smoking-and-cancer (2015)

6   See oxygen.org.au/images/Australian_Bureau_of_Statistics_Smoking_Prevalence_2007-08.pdf (2015)

7   From en.wikipedia.org/wiki/Smoking_in_Germany (2015)

smokers.[8]

The above Wikipedia article says "In Chinese culture, smoking is connected to masculine identity as a social activity that is practiced among men to promote feelings of acceptance and brotherhood"[9]. That would be the effect of advertising, surely, not simply a "cultural" matter.

In English-speaking western countries where smoking rates are relatively low, there is a perception that the problem is under control. Still, about one in five or six adults smoke and smoking is still killing millions of people even in the countries where anti-smoking legislation is most aggressive. That one in five or six adults still smoke in the USA, Canada, England, and Australia is surprising, given that smoking is now mainly a furtive outdoor activity that is banned from all indoor public places. Moreover, tobacco advertising is severely limited in these countries.

> In Canada, the advertising of tobacco products was prohibited by the Tobacco Products Control Act as of 1988[10].

How do tobacco companies still manage to hook one in five adults? They introduce new products such as e-cigarettes that may not be regulated by legislation for some time. They introduce fruity flavorings that especially appeal to children. They sponsor events. They pay movie producers for their products to appear in movies. The internet has created a vast new zone for marketing. They work youtube.com and other such media sites. They spend millions wriggling in the loopholes they exploit to market their products to youngsters[11].

The smoking rates for youth in Canada are the same as among adults.

---

8   From en.wikipedia.org/wiki/Smoking_in_China (2015). See also economist.com/news/china/21597958-smoking-course-kill-100m-chinese-people-century-will-latest-anti-smoking (2015)

9   Ibid.

10 From en.wikipedia.org/wiki/Tobacco_advertising#Canada (2015)

11 See theglobeandmail.com/life/health-and-fitness/health/e-cigarettes-could-hook-a-new-generation-on-nicotine-experts-warn/article14740075 (2015) for an example of wriggle.

This is not surprising: the youths emulate the adults in this sort of behavior.

Tobacco companies are not allowed to but do target youth. Most smokers start as teenagers. It's not a decision adults will make so often. How do tobacco companies target youth? The research of Pamela Ling and Stanton Glantz[12] indicates considerable tobacco-industry research into the cultivation of youth and turning them into regular smokers over the course of stages and years.

12 See "Why and How the Tobacco Industry Sells Cigarettes to Young Adults: Evidence From Industry Documents", Pamela Ling, Stanton Glantz, ncbi.nlm.nih.gov/pmc/articles/PMC1447481 (2015).

24 - Smoking and Stress Reduction

You may feel that smoking gives you things in your life that you treasure. The reason that smokers don't stop is because they are convinced they can't have those things without smoking, or not as fully without smoking.

They think that stopping has to be a terrible experience because that's what it has been in the past when they've tried, usually with a method that requires much willpower.

Once you understand what it is you think smoking gives you that is of importance to you, it's important to examine very carefully whether smoking *actually gives you that thing or things*. The answer is going to be an extremely emphatic "No, it doesn't give you those things. You supply them yourself, and you always have. All smoking gives you is a blood sucker on your neck."

For instance, many people believe that smoking helps them deal with stress. And of course dealing with stress is something we all have to be able to do. Some more than others. And often heavy smokers are people in positions requiring heavy stress management. Perhaps like King George VI. The idea of not being able to deal with the stress they have to deal with constantly is scary.

What smoking contributes to managing stress is this: *more stress*, not less. And here's why. Smoking provides the illusion of helping with stress by providing two things: stressful withdrawal symptoms and, when you smoke, temporary cessation of the withdrawal symptoms. Smoking doesn't do anything to alleviate stress caused by other considerations, like whether the Nazis are going to conquer England, if you're King George VI. Smoking only alleviates stress caused by nicotine addiction. But it also causes that stress. It's a self-perpetuating stressor. People who stop smoking find that their stress levels *decrease*. Smoking is an *additional* stressful burden, not something that decreases stress.

People who treasure smoking because they think it helps them manage stress have to give *themselves* some credit for managing the stress in their lives. They manage that stress themselves! Cigarettes don't help at all. All this time, *you* have been fully sufficient to the job of managing stress. And have even been managing more stress than you need to because smoking just causes more stress.

Nicotine is a stimulant. It makes your heart pound. It causes adrenaline levels to rise. That is the "fight or flight" hormone. This is not relaxing at all. It's stressful. However, the nicotine alleviates the nicotine withdrawal symptoms.

If you're the type of person who treasures smoking to manage stress, then when you understand that smoking does not help you deal with stress and that you yourself have been the one successfully managing your stress, a seemingly magical thing happens. You no longer feel urges to smoke. You are freed from that torment. Completely. Enjoyably. Fully. Joyously.

Why? Because those urges are 99% psychological. Those urges were a manifestation of your fears and insecurities about what was stressing you. When you understand that smoking was merely a stressor, not a stress reducer, you understand that you don't need to smoke to manage stress. And the urges simply disappear.

What you have, instead, is confidence that you yourself are capable of managing the stress. And that is real confidence. Putting confidence in cigarettes is not real confidence. It's the result of a confidence trick that tobacco companies have played on you. They count on you thinking you need cigarettes to do the job of managing stress. They rely on your insecurities to turn you into a reliable addict customer of theirs, virtually a slave of theirs, paying them every day for the poison, lies and illusions they dispense.

All this time, it's you who have dealt with your stress successfully. Smoking never helped you with it one little bit. You've been giving it credit it does not deserve. Give yourself the credit you deserve. You are up to the job. *The proof is that you've been doing it all this time on your own*—with the added burden of a smoking addiction causing more stress.

25 - Brainwashing

We think of 'brainwashing' as something out of The Manchurian Candidate. In that 1959 film, USAmerican soldiers are captured by the Chinese and brainwashed into attempting to assassinate the President.

It's a Hollywood film. The notion of brainwashing it presents seems about as likely to exist as Godzilla or King Kong. We suspect no one can control somebody else's mind to the extent that they can be made to do something like a political assassination against their own will.

I smoked for thirty years. That's a long time. The main things that kept me smoking all those years were illusions about what it was doing for me, the illusion that life wouldn't be as good without it. The feeling that I needed to smoke was real. But I didn't really need it.

So it seems I was brainwashed for thirty years, brainwashed and complicit in my own brainwashing. I didn't question my illusions about smoking. I didn't question whether it was giving me what I thought it was giving me, and I thought that the addiction was mainly chemical, not psychological.

What started out as an 'aide' for a teenager to be an adult eventually turned into an 'aide' for a young man to be an artist, a writer. I see better now how smoking addressed my basic fears and insecurities about being a man, about being a creative artist, about being able to cope with stress. But, also, my parents smoked and so did many of my friends; it was an unquestioned, ever-present part of life.

We don't change what we don't question. If we don't question something about ourselves, it probably isn't going to change; we won't be the ones doing it, if it does. Socrates said that the unexamined life is not worth living. Because it's the life of a zombie.

The basic proposition in brainwashing is often that our insecurities will be assuaged by doing what the brainwashing suggests we do. The basic proposition is that we are weak, afraid, and in need of a crutch.

That is not unique to how cigarettes are marketed. Cosmetics, deodorants, clothing, hair loss products, acne cream, erection pills, on and on...these products play on peoples' insecurities that they are *inadequate* in some way that the product redresses. Some of these products do actually help you with something. But the marketing plays on peoples' fears nonetheless. Cigarettes are marketed like many other products—but they are different in that the product does *nothing* for you, is physically addictive, and is highly toxic. The marketing for all the above products seeks to put you under the illusion that the product does more for you than it actually does.

26 - Brainwashing and Revolution

When you stop smoking, your perspective on 'brainwashing' changes. It's a time of wonder and reflection. When I stopped smoking after thirty years, I had to wonder how it was that I remained brainwashed for such a long time. And was it my own doing? It's easy to stop once you examine and dispel the illusions you maintain about what smoking gives you. Once those illusions are dispelled, the psychological dependency is almost finished. In the light of day, we wonder how such apparently weak illusions could hold us for so long in such a deadly embrace. How were the weak illusions that strong, that enduring?

Definitions of 'brainwashing' in dictionaries show us two apparently quite different meanings. The first meaning of 'brainwashing' describes it as "a forcible indoctrination to induce someone to give up basic political, social, or religious beliefs and attitudes and to accept contrasting regimented ideas" (Merriam-Webster). The idea is that it's *forcible*, against the person's will. The second meaning is that 'brainwashing' is "persuasion by propaganda or salesmanship" (Merriam-Webster). There is a world of difference between these two definitions. The second one doesn't have the *forcible* dimension to it. It's not even necessarily a face-to-face encounter.

My own brainwashing about smoking, brainwashing that kept me smoking for thirty years, was not forcible. I became a smoker because I wanted to emulate my parents and be an adult myself. Smoking was an adult thing I could do when I was not yet an adult. I was curious about addiction, also. I doubted that I could be addicted to cigarettes, and wanted to know how addiction worked.

Once I started smoking and of course didn't like it, I hoped to acquire a taste for it because I thought that acquiring such a taste was a sign of being adult. Adults, I thought, appreciate such strong assaults upon the senses. Perhaps it makes you feel truly alive, I thought.

I used to steal from my mother's cigarettes. And I think there was a kind of sexual connection with my mother going on in my smoking. I stole her cigarettes, smoked hers, experienced her experience of intoxication with cigarettes vicariously, the unfiltered Buckinghams. We were 'smoking together' as it were.

Smoking always retained a twisted romance and solidarity for me with my parents, both of whom I loved dearly, being their only offspring. We all smoked. They both died of it and smoked nearly to the end.

My dad tried stopping several times. One time we were doing well at it together but I relapsed. He wasn't far behind. I felt guilty about starting up again and ruining it for him. Because he needed to stop more than I did.

It's often the case that smokers are in a group of smokers of some sort, whether it's family or at work or with friends. The "peace pipe" is a relatively early well-known example of bonding by smoking. Something done together between people.

My addiction was formed in relation to my parents in a desire to be like them and to be an adult with them. I didn't think of it as self-destructive. I viewed it as an adult pleasure. As I became a regular smoker, I thought of it as an aide to concentration, relaxation, stress management, and the like.

The notion that it's a confidence game based on illusions was not something I would have entertained. And the notion that my parents had fallen for such a deception would have been scary and offensive to me. They were not dupes. They were my wise and loving parents.

Well, yes, they were dupes, but so was I for 30 years. And so was/is a sizable portion of the entire population. It isn't a matter of being stupid or a sucker. Yes, duped, but falling into the confidence trick not out of greed or arrogance or stupidity but fundamentally out of insecurity and not feeling confident enough to be able to handle everything that comes one's way without a bit of help. That's human. It's out of vulnerability and insecurity. It's out of a fear that we can't handle things on our own and need a bit of help. And it's out of wanting to be part of a group of people we admire or love or work among, need acceptance from.

The enticement to be an adult obviously doesn't motivate an adult. Instead, young adults are offered different enticements. Like the notion that smoking will help them cope with the adult world and its new and scary challenges. This is when the notion that it helps with concentration, relaxation etc., becomes attractive.

The things that attract children to smoking are different from the things that keep them coming back as adults. Tobacco companies know this deeply[13]. However, while the machinations of tobacco companies influence our own brainwashing, the biggest factor is us. We ourselves. In their song "Revolution," the Beatles say:

> You say you'll change the constitution
> Well, you know
> We all want to change your head.
> You tell me it's the institution
> Well, you know
> You'd better free your mind instead.

The key to stopping smoking is freeing your own mind from illusions about what smoking is doing for you. Once you start questioning what smoking is really doing for you, once you start thinking about it in your daily life, the unquestioned has become the questioned, and those illusions are not long for this world. Illusions do well in the dark. Once you start thinking about them and recognize and understand them as illusions, once you shine some light on them, they don't last long.

Stopping smoking is always an important revolution in the life of whoever stops smoking. It's not simply a matter of breaking a deadly addiction. It's a matter of freeing your mind from falsehoods, illusions. That's enjoyable. And a relief. Acknowledging the truth is always a relief. Denial is painful and difficult.

Stopping smoking is enjoyable in many ways. One of them is the sense of achievement, of doing something that you wanted to do for a long time. There is also a sense of enjoyment and satisfaction coming to a deeper, useful understanding of the mechanism of the addiction to smoking. And you understand yourself better. You understand what you thought smoking was giving you, and you will understand that it doesn't give you those things—you give them to yourself. You can't easily fool yourself anymore about the notion that you enjoyed smoking, or that you need one to relax or concentrate. You know yourself a bit better.

Stopping smoking gives you the enjoyment of the seeker. The seeker

---

13 See "Why and How the Tobacco Industry Sells Cigarettes to Young Adults: Evidence From Industry Documents", Pamela Ling, Stanton Glantz, ncbi.nlm.nih.gov/pmc/articles/PMC1447481 (2015).

after truth. The truth is that the urge to smoke is mainly psychological. It needs you to be under the sway of illusions that amplify the twinges of hunger for nicotine into urges. Once those illusions are dispelled, you fully and completely understand you don't need to smoke to get what you need.

Once you really know this to be true—and you'll know it to be true because you no longer desire to smoke—the urges are gone—you feel a bit like the seeker in The Flammarion engraving who has discovered the Empyrean beyond the stars.

Who would unknow what they have come to know? Especially when that knowledge is hard-won? Once you know the truth of the urge to smoke, you will never forget it.

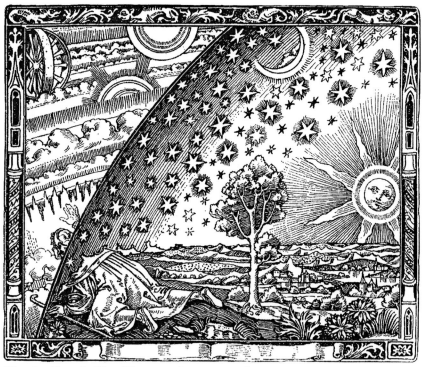

Illustration 1: The Flammarion engraving

27 - Brainwashing and Denial

Whether we call it brainwashing or something else, smokers engage in a horrendously damaging activity, often for decades or even until it kills them, and don't feel that it's in their power to stop even though just about all smokers would like to stop. Smokers aren't coerced/brainwashed into shooting the President—that is the brainwashing in The Manchurian Candidate—but many smokers end up killing themselves by smoking as surely as if they'd put a bullet in their own head.

We can become so *invested* in our smoking that changing our attitudes and thoughts about it can seem like an admission of error and defeat, an admission of having lived improperly, an admission of having thrown it all away for nothing.

When my dad was dying of lung cancer, all the care givers in the house were smokers, including me. And we were all still smoking in the house. He, of course, was experiencing breathing difficulties. I told him we would all stop smoking in the house. He said no. As though it was an article of freedom. "We're not going to stop smoking," he said. He wouldn't have us unfree to smoke in the house. He asked me to buy a couple of air filters.

The poor man. With three smoking care givers. And he smoked right up till the end. He was too invested in it to contemplate such a change. And we were too plain-old addicted to do the obvious thing: take it outside.

Sometimes we maintain our illusions out of pride and a sense that we would sacrifice our dignity if we relinquished our illusions. But dad always valued the truth. Or thought he did. Until it seemed too painful to face, in this case.

He was very far from a coward, though. He once risked death, when no one else who was there would, to pull some people out of a fire at a head-on car accident. People were shouting to him to get out of there. It *did* explode not long after he got out, having saved a boy. He was my hero. And not just for that. He was a very fine man. He was brave to save others the day he pulled those people out of a burning wreck.

Funny thing, though: however painful it seems to face the truth, not facing it ends up being more painful.

Neither of the definitions of brainwashing in the dictionary talk about our own role in our own brainwashing. Whether the ideas/beliefs in the brainwashing process are forced on us or not, we ourselves are the ones who keep ourselves believing in the reality of our illusions.

To keep an open mind is to remain open to the possibility that we have deluded ourselves for a very long time. To admit that possibility is not to admit that one has thrown one's life away or lived improperly. *It's simply to admit that we are human and subject to illusions. We are vulnerable, we are subject to error, we are imperfect, we are human. And to admit it and to keep an open mind is to value the truth.* To value the truth enough to admit we have treasured our illusions too fearfully is a great relief. A great relief from the suffering of sustained denial. And it opens the way to healing, to positive change.

It's never too late to discover the truth. Only the truth will set us free. Even lovers of truth, such as my father truly was, can be trapped in denial. What a relief it would have been for him to have been able to put aside smoking at the end. I wish I could have helped him with that.

His death was a terrifying experience for me. He was not ready to go. He didn't want to go and he didn't want to deal with his denial about smoking. For him, stopping smoking was to stop being able to enjoy life. Right up to the end. That's a hard way to go.

28 - Smoking and Boredom

One sometimes hears that smokers smoke when they're bored, to relieve boredom. That's similar to something I heard from a smoker who described his as a "hand to mouth addiction." He was convinced he was addicted to moving his hand to his mouth. I suggested that, instead, he was addicted to the smoking he was able to do once he got his hand (with a cigarette in it) to his mouth. A good test of this would be to move his hand (without a cigarette in it) to his mouth.

What smoking relieves is nicotine withdrawal, not boredom. Smokers smoke when they're bored because it presents a convenient opportunity to relieve the discomfort of nicotine withdrawal. It isn't simply a matter of smoking providing something to do when bored. Smoking is not an exciting or even an enjoyable activity. But it does temporarily relieve withdrawal symptoms of nicotine addiction. That is why smokers smoke when they are bored.

When you stop smoking, you will not be drawn to smoke when you are bored. For most people, periods when they have no demands on them are productive times of reflection and relaxation. During such times, you won't want a cigarette. It would be an unwelcome interruption and destructive of all that you do want.

But those aren't times of boredom. Boredom is when we have no demands on us but are unable to engage in reflection and relaxation. Boredom is aimless Jonesing. Some irritation is preventing us from enjoying our down-time. For smokers, that irritation is often nicotine withdrawal. For others, it's anxiety of some sort. For smokers, it's anxiety *amplified* by nicotine withdrawal into urges to smoke.

Smoking is often misconstrued as a useful way to deal with anxiety. But it merely increases one's anxiety. Nicotine withdrawal is discomfort that causes anxiety. Smoking may temporarily relieve that anxiety, but it also ensures future discomfort and anxiety: the withdrawal discomfort will soon start again. Additionally, smoking causes other anxieties. You worry about what smoking is doing to your health and what it's doing to your relationships, for instance.

There will be less stress and anxiety when you stop smoking. And less boredom, because boredom is when you are anxious and scattered.

29 - Substitutes

Some methods of stopping smoking substitute one form of nicotine for another. Such as patches or gum or now e-cigarettes. But you still have an addiction to nicotine. And a psychological dependence on smoking. You, however, are not going to need any substitutes. Because we get rid of your desire to smoke.

You don't need a substitute for something you don't want.

Addiction to cigarettes is primarily a psychological matter. Consequently, nicotine substitutes do not cure an addiction but transfer it to another nicotine product.

I tried nicotine gum. I ended up chewing it for three years. But eventually went back to smoking. Because I still desired cigarettes. I hadn't dealt with my addiction. I'd simply transferred it to chewing gum. I was still a nicotine addict and I was still under the illusion that I needed nicotine.

Once those illusions are dispelled, you know you don't need nicotine in any form whatsoever for anything.

Substitutes take addicts down another garden path. Yes it's typically a less harmful path because gums and patches probably are not as bad for you as smoking. But most people end up smoking again.

These methods throw a pill—or a patch or a gum—at a problem that a pill won't cure. What cures the problem is dealing with the addiction, not transferring it to a different product.

Some careful thought, reflection, and meditation goes a long way. Some self-knowledge. Self-knowledge is more transformative than a pill.

The permanent cure for smoking is understanding and dispelling the illusions we have about what smoking is supposedly giving us but really isn't at all. Without that understanding, those illusions still have their power over us and we transfer our real need for the things we think smoking gives us into cravings for cigarettes—or patches, gums, etc. Cravings are a result of the double physical plus psychological dependence. The physical dependence of addiction to nicotine sets up the cycle of drug taking and then withdrawal symptoms.

30 - My Experience With Zyban

The first time I stopped smoking, I used Zyban, otherwise known as Wellbutrin, a popular 'anti-smoking' drug that is an anti-depressant. Coincidentally, the woman I was seeing, at the time, was using Wellbutrin as an anti-depressant. When I read the literature on my package of Zyban, it said not to use Wellbutrin with Zyban. I was surprised to learn that they are exactly the same thing with different names. I had never taken an anti-depressant before. I was surprised to learn that I now was. And of course it was a little um funny that my girlfriend and I were both taking the same anti-depressant under different names for quite different reasons.

There were several problems with my first attempt to stop smoking. First and foremost, I was stopping because the woman I was seeing asked me to, not primarily because I wanted to. That, in itself, is enough to doom the attempt to stop smoking.

But, secondly, I was attempting to use a pill for something that requires more mindfulness than a pill solely can provide. A pill does not, on its own, dismantle the psychological dependence. If the psychological addiction is not dismantled, it will be a problem.

What the Zyban pill does is take the edge off of anxiety. That's what my girlfriend was taking it for. Urges to smoke are mainly made of fear, anxiety and/or other emotions transferred and amplified into an urge to smoke. Smoking is how smokers believe they allay anxiety, fear, sadness, and other emotions. Zyban takes the edge off of anxiety, so it makes for less strong urges to smoke.

The Zyban literature instructed me to think about the situations that triggered my urges to smoke, and to prepare some alternatives or substitute to smoking for those occasions or to figure out ways to avoid or minimize those situations. So I went to a great toy store and got some fun puzzles and toys to play with in situations where I got an urge to smoke, for instance.

Looking back, I see that while minimizing the 'trigger' experiences and planning substitute activities is indeed useful—and I advise you do so—these are stop-gap measures if one does not dismantle one's psychological addiction. The urges may continue after having stopped taking Zyban.

I also had problems with withdrawal from Zyban. I wasn't suicidal, but my mind was a little darker and out of my control than is normally the case, for me. It was a little trepidatious for a couple of weeks or a month.

When I stopped taking Zyban at the prescribed time, I had successfully abstained from smoking since I started the drug. So far so good. And I didn't have a cigarette until not long after the romance with my girlfriend ended. The romance with her was over but the romance with smoking was not.

By all means, consider the situations that give rise to your urges for a cigarette and think of alternative activities for those situations and also minimize those situations, when possible. For instance, if you normally have a cigarette after a meal, substitute some other activity that you enjoy instead of smoking. Or if you normally smoke when you drink, don't drink or drink something other than alcohol. Or if you smoke when you read or concentrate, get something to keep your hands busy when you concentrate. If you smoke by rewarding yourself, create a different awards system. Breathing exercises are useful sometimes, such as when you want to concentrate or when stress, anxiety, worry, fear, or other such states of mind occur. We'll talk more about breathing and breathing exercises.

But keep in mind that you are hooked when you want a cigarette. You are simply landed when you have one. *You don't need a substitute for something you don't want.* If you don't want a cigarette, if you feel no urge to smoke, then you don't need any substitutes for smoking. The idea is to get rid of your desires/urges to smoke, not simply find ways to successfully suffer through them when they occur.

Still, there are going to be occasions when you want one, even if you successfully dismantle your psychological dependence. These wants won't be as urgent as when you smoked, but you will sometimes have to deal with desires to smoke, for a while.

I sometimes even get a kind of a lust for a cigarette. But it isn't an abiding thing. It's gone as quickly as it comes. It doesn't have the power it used to have over me. It is as an illusion that briefly rises to consciousness and soon disappears under the waves. I am not under the illusion that feeding my occasional desire for a cigarette will bring me any satisfaction. I realize that smoking does not give me the things I thought it gave me. And I can call on my joy in being a non-smoker. I can laugh about it. Smoking involves taking some illusions more seriously than they should be taken.

But, still, I need to be careful. It does not pay to think that you are beyond being controlled by addiction. That would indicate a kind of arrogant pride that would result in your thinking you can smoke without falling into regular use.

I can see how Zyban might be useful to some people because it takes the edge off of anxiety. However, just by itself it isn't going to be sufficient. It does nothing to dismantle the psychological dependence. If you take Zyban to help you stop smoking, read the instructions very carefully, talk with a doctor, and read online about the experience of other people with it. Such drugs, while possibly helpful, can create their own set of problems. And get help dismantling the psychological addiction.

A drug to take the edge off of anxiety and fear can conceivably be useful to some people. However, it's important to come to an understanding of the relation of your fear and anxiety to smoking. Many people think that smoking helps them deal with their fear and anxiety. It's crucial to fully understand that smoking does not help but, instead, hurts you even in these regards.

31 - Breathe Deeply

If you read stories or watch films, notice how many of them start with the main character experiencing a departure from his/her usual routine. In fiction and in life, that's when things get interesting. You are at such a juncture. Stopping smoking is a departure from your routine. Departures are sometimes exciting and interesting. The zest of life is in such shake-ups of the status quo. They present lively challenges and new perspectives, new vistas.

Some people wait till their holidays to stop smoking so that they're not under much stress but also so that they can be in a foreign environment where their routine is not asserting that it's time for a smoke at all the regular times, events and places.

It's good to try new things when you stop smoking to break up the routine. So that your 'trigger events' are not as frequent or in the same context. So that they're somehow different. But you can do that whether you're on holidays or at home—and you're eventually going to have to do it at home *anyway*.

Breathing exercises aren't simply a boring exercise in sighing plaintively. They're an exciting addition to your life that can change your life in fantastic ways. That's what we're going to talk about this chapter.

Smoking is the worst possible breathing exercise, of course, apart from no breathing at all. But smokers, when smoking, typically breathe somewhat deeply. That activity—*without smoking*—is beneficial and pleasing. When you take a deep breath of fresh air, feel the muscles in your chest; feel how they respond to your deep breath. They like it. Particularly at the moment when you reach the top of your breath. The muscles stretch a bit, and stretching muscles feels good. Deep, slow breathing is relaxing and energizing. Take a breath and hold it briefly, then exhale. How does that feel to the chest muscles? A bit different than not holding the deep breath. Both are good.

Singers, prior to a performance, typically do breathing exercises before they start their vocal exercises. The breathing exercises get the muscles ready for the show and start tuning up the pipes. Breathing exercises also prepare the spirit for singing. *Breathing exercises make you feel good*—your spirit leaves the ground like a bird jumping into the air. It's uplifting.

The English word *spirit* is from the Latin *spiritus* which means *breath*. Breath and spirit, by definition, are linked. Your spirit moves with your breath. What that means is how you feel has a lot to do with how you breathe and how you breathe has a lot to do with how you feel. You can make yourself feel better by taking deep breaths and exploring other breathing exercises.

The word *inspiration* refers to drawing air into the lungs. To breathe deeply is *inspiring*. Breathing-in is a life-sustaining act—we can't live without breathing—and there is a kind of pleasure at the top of each breath we draw, a pleasure in receiving the oxygen that sustains us from moment to moment. At the top of a breath—the first moment when our lungs are full—it feels like there's an oxygen feeding frenzy going on in our lungs; our body revels in that brief moment of *literal inspiration* when the oxygen in the lungs is being extracted and the tissue is slightly stretched from full lungs; we are *infused* with precious oxygen. Each breath is a meal of oxygen for the lungs and is devoured hungrily, resulting for a brief moment, at the top of the breath, in pleasure and relief, the same sort of pleasure and relief we get from a meal when we are hungry, only much briefer and more subtle, and there is also the pleasure of stretching, at that moment, if the breath is deep. Take a deep breath and hold it for a moment before exhaling. *That is the feeling of inspiration.*

Value that pleasure and relief at the top of a full breath of fresh air, appreciate it, be grateful for it. That is indeed the infusion of our bodies with "life force" and an *inspiration* to treasure.

Breathing isn't built into the word "spirit" or "inspiration" by accident. Good breathing exercises/techniques are important to meditation and spirituality and have been since ancient times. When we are anxious, afraid, or tense, our breathing tends to be shallow and fast. When we are happy, our breathing is deeper and slower. When we feel a certain way, we tend to breathe a certain way. But it is also possible to *change how we feel by breathing differently.* Good breathing actually changes how we are feeling emotionally/spiritually.

The Sanskrit word *prana* means "life force" or "vital principle"—or "breath". In Hindu philosophy, *prana* is the essence of life permeating the universe. The 3,000 year-old Chandogya Upanishad is one of our earliest references to *prana*. It's an important idea in yoga, Indian medicine, and martial arts. This concept migrated to China as Ch'i and later to Japan, where it is named Ki.

If we think of the essence of life, well, what is it, and how would ancients think of it? What sort of properties does it have? Surely it can *move*. Movement is important to living things.

> Prana is typically divided into multiple constituent parts, in particular when concerned with the human body. While not all early sources agree on the names or number of these subdivisions, the most common list from the Mahabharata, the Upanishads, Ayurvedic and Yogic sources includes five, often divided into further subcategories. This list includes: Prana (inward moving energy), Apana (outward moving energy), Vyana (circulation of energy), Udana (energy of the head and throat), and Samana (digestion and assimilation). Early mention of specific pranas often emphasized Prāṇa Apāna and Vyāna as "the three breaths".[14]

Prana, as it relates to the human body, is presented as *energy flow*. Which very much involves the breath (intake and expulsion of air), as well as intake and expulsion of food and liquid—and of course intake and expulsion of information. Breathing is central to our health. If we don't breath, we're in trouble.

So, going back to ancient times, breathing has been linked to "spirit" and "life force". Breathing can be a source of great energy. Deep breathing of fresh air is so vitalizing, so fundamentally linked not only to survival but to the full appreciation and enjoyment of being alive that the very definitions of "inspiration" and the "life force", the cosmic energy of the universe, are directly linked to breathing.

> Prāṇāyāma...is a Sanskrit word meaning "extension of the prāṇa or breath" or "extension of the life force". The word is composed from two Sanskrit words: prana meaning life force (noted particularly as the breath), and ayāma, to extend or draw out. (Not

---

14 See en.wikipedia.org/wiki/Prana

"restrain, or control" as is often translated from yam instead of ayāma). It is a yogic discipline with origins in ancient India.[15]

Pranayama is associated with breathing exercises for relaxation, concentration, and other health benefits. If you Google "Kundalini Yoga Pranayama" you will encounter many useful breathing exercises. Youtube has lots of instructive videos on the matter.

You don't have to become a yogi or get religion for this to work for you. The basic idea is that you can manage stress, relaxation, and concentration with simple breathing exercises *much better than through smoking.*

It's interesting to learn that George Lucas, the creator of Star Wars, seems to have gotten his idea for "the force," at least in part, from *prana.* We read in Wikipedia that "The natural flow of energy known as The Force is believed to have originated from the concept of prana, or qi/chi/ki, "the all-pervading vital energy of the universe".[16] Though it should be added that Lucas's "the force" seems also to involve related but different notions from different cultures.[17] Lucas took a consciously cross-cultural approach to re-telling old myths in new ways in Star Wars.

Taking up breathing exercises may not turn you into a Jedi Knight capable of moving objects with your mind, but it just might change your life for the better. It'll help you relax, focus, concentrate, and value your breath, your breathing as an instrument of vigor and vitality.

There are other pleasures, surprises, consolations, delights and even inspirations that await you in your exploration of the seemingly simple act of breathing which open up to you as you stop smoking. If you've never explored the ways you can breathe and how they make you feel, check them out. But don't pass out. The goal here is to find what makes you *feel good,* not simply to try everything out like a maniac. Keep in mind that if you breathe rapidly for too long, you will hyper-ventilate and pass out. Don't do that. See how breathing

15 See en.wikipedia.org/wiki/Pranayama

16 See en.wikipedia.org/wiki/Star_Wars_sources_and_analogues

17 See starwars.wikia.com/wiki/The_Force for an interesting discussion of "the force" in Star Wars.

differently makes you feel—because breath and spirit are indeed linked.

What is most relaxing are deep easy breaths. Breathe in deeply and exhale slowly, easily, with little effort twenty times. How does that feel? You should actually feel your spirit lift in this simple act. Take a short break and then do it twenty more times.

It isn't addictive! The difference between what's involved in taking up breathing as part of your regimen and taking up smoking is interesting. You have to cultivate breathing techniques and exercises consciously and continually choose things. You're never addicted. It's always about conscious choices even though you have to keep breathing to keep living.

Breathing exercises and regimens help some people get rid of their asthma via the Buteyko breathing techniques. These techniques promise to help you unplug your nose and breathe better at night, also. If you breathe through your mouth a lot, it's possible to easily learn how to breathe through your nose 24/7. Learning to breathe through your nose 24/7, even during exercise, has health benefits including less phlegm and better oxygen absorption.

When you stop smoking, it isn't long before you don't wheeze anymore. Your breathing gets deeper, too; your lung capacity increases. Breathing exercises increase it even more. You are going to get a high-performance set of lungs good for lots of exercise, much more singing than you could do while you were a smoker, and the real pleasure of breathing fresh air. And your new high-performance lungs will let you breathe in ways that allow you to regulate your stress/concentration/mood much better than smoking ever did.

But breathing exercises don't dismantle psychological dependence on smoking. Breathing exercises are very useful to you in situations where you want to smoke, but it doesn't get to the root of the urge to smoke.

So your breathing exercises should be different from your breathing when you smoke. Your breathing exercises should involve types of breathing that aren't very easy for smokers to do, so that you value being a non-smoker. A simple succession of deep, easy, slow breaths will suffice, most of the time. This isn't even conspicuous. You can do it in the subway.

Another type of breathing exercise good for people who have stopped smoking is this. Take a deep breath and slowly exhale. Then take a slightly deeper breath and hold it briefly. Then slowly exhale. Take slightly ever-deeper breaths, holding them ever-slightly longer, until you begin to experience discomfort. Then stop and take a few short, easy breaths. You should feel lighter and more relaxed. This also helps you increase your lung capacity, which will continue for years after you stop smoking.

Please take an active interest in figuring out how to reduce stress by deep breathing. It isn't hard. See how deep breathing makes you feel better, relaxes you, energizes you—delights you.

The experience should contrast with smoking. What you don't want is for your breathing exercises to make you feel like smoking. When you stop smoking, you gain the ability to do things you couldn't do, or couldn't do so easily or joyfully, as when you smoked. It's good to take advantage of those new abilities—not only because they themselves are positive and healthy, but because it helps you *value* being a non-smoker. You can do things that become important to you that you can't do as a smoker. That helps you stay off smoking, so you can do them.

Luckily, good deep breathing is quite unlike what one does while smoking. Breathing when smoking usually isn't as deep or as regular. You take a puff and then breathe less deeply for a while. Whereas good deep breathing involves an uninterrupted succession of several deep breaths. You don't have to huff and puff. Just a few deep, easy breaths followed by slow, easy, shallower breathing for a while. Then a few more successive deep breaths, and so on.

Also, the result of good deep breathing is different from smoking. You feel energized, not stupefied. Your spirits are lifted. Your brain is oxygenated/fed and clear. It's better than drugs and it's 100% natural you. No accessories required.

Stopping smoking gives you the opportunity to turn breathing into something that infuses you with energy rather than something that poisons you. Rather than having your breathing co-opted and corrupted by smoking, you are now in a position to learn about how to breathe so that you have more control over your spiritual/emotional/intellectual state. Smoking hands that control over to tobacco because your breathing is regulated by the limitations it imposes on you. Smokers tend not to explore their breathing very much and might even think that idea is odd—a wee bit freaky and off limits. Little do they realize that's because their breath is being stolen from them. It's very uncool for smokers to look at what their breathing can do for them without smoking. Why is it so uncool? Because one good look at what breathing can offer you without smoking is dramatic enough to make you want to stop smoking.

To explore your breathing is to explore your spirit. Not to explore your breathing is to give up an ancient and important way to regulate your emotional/spiritual/intellectual being. If you can't learn to value and treasure the infusion of your body with life force via breathing fresh air deeply, you deny yourself the health, vitality and *inspiration* you deserve as a human being.

So explore it like the captain of a new ship in a new world. Sail that ship where you have not gone before. The wind is high; the cheeks of Zephyrus filled with propitious breath.

The Indian word for breath exercises that extend, expand, move, and increase your life force is *pranayama*. What you come to understand is that part of the reliance smokers have on smoking is that it becomes a terrible alternative for breathing exercises. Breathing exercises are *magnificently superior* to smoking as ways to relieve stress, achieve peace of mind and concentration, acceptance of yourself, and enjoyment of life. Your spirit and your breath are indeed linked. Explore that link with your new-found freedom to do so. You will find it keenly pleasurable and rewarding.

But breathing exercises do not satisfy urges to smoke. They're not a substitute for smoking, though they may calm or even get rid of urges sometimes. Urges to smoke are mainly a matter of psychological addiction. Dismantling your psychological addiction gets rid of urges to smoke. Breathing exercises open up a whole different way to enjoy your body, your life, and regulate your moods, concentration and energy.

32 - The Mythos of Smoking

It isn't widely known that it isn't difficult to get rid of the urges for cigarettes. So that you don't have to wage an epic battle of willpower to stop smoking. Once the urges disappear, stopping smoking gets a lot easier. It isn't very widely known that it's relatively easy to get rid of the urges. This contradicts the whole *mythos* of smoking.

A *mythos* is a set of beliefs or assumptions about something. Many of the items of the mythos of smoking are false. Such as that smoking tastes good, that it's a stress reducer, a concentration aide, a weight loss aide, a relaxant, that it makes you more adult, makes you cool, makes you one of the crowd. Another falsity is that it's very difficult to stop smoking. All those falsehoods are enticements to smoke or to remain smoking.

The idea that the addiction is 99% psychological is not part of the general knowledge about smoking, is not part of the mythos. Instead, most people think that the addiction is mainly chemical, that the cause of the strong urges smokers experience is primarily chemical. But that is false.

One of the main things that makes stopping smoking so difficult is the misinformation we believe about smoking. It's so prominent in society. Why isn't the truth more prominent? I think it's at least partly because so much money is made from smokers. There's far more money involved in keeping people hooked than in helping them ditch the poison.

Currently (2016), in most western nations, about 16-20% of the adult population smokes. The numbers are much higher in many other places. China has more than 300 million smokers and more than half of Chinese male adults smoke. In any case, the money involved, whether we're talking about China—or even Canada—is gargantuan.

In Canada in 2012, 16% of the adult population smoked. In the USA in 2012, 18.1% of the adult population smoked. There were about 35 million Canadians, in total, in 2012. If we say that the average smoker smokes a pack a day, and a pack in Canada costs, on average, $10, then Canadians spent $56 million per day on cigarettes in 2012.

That's an extraordinary amount of money even in a country with a small population. That money mainly goes to different levels of government and to the cigarette companies. Governments are hooked on tobacco revenues. They are invested, and have been for several hundred years.

But they also want smokers to quit because smokers get expensive and need all sorts of health care that non-smokers don't typically need. There's a whole industry around medical treatments to stop smoking, mainly via nicotine replacements. Which don't cure the addiction but transfer it to another expensive substance. You don't smoke anymore but you're still a reliable addict customer.

There's another industry in treating the diseases from smoking. There's an industry to provide cigarettes, another one to 'help' with the addiction and another one to provide medical treatments for the diseases it causes.

The blood suckers are just *so thick and numerous* in all of this that there is *little room for the truth*. The truth is that there is a much easier, simpler, permanent cure for tobacco addiction than is widely understood.

Smokers get feasted on by tobacco companies, government, and, eventually, the health care industry. The tobacco companies hook you with a confidence game and the government and medical establishments are as hooked on tobacco revenues as smokers themselves are on nicotine.

And that's another thing that makes smoking so hard to stop. There are so many businesses invested in the myth of it being hard to stop that it remains a mainly unchallenged part of the mythos of smoking. There are significant and numerous long-standing, powerful interests in the idea that it's very hard to disengage from nicotine consumption.

The truth that the addiction is 99% psychological and the urges can be eliminated by dispelling some illusions is not in the public mind as widely as the idea that a pill or gum might do the trick.

It takes some doing to stay a non-smoker even after you've dismantled the psychological addiction, but it isn't a torturous ordeal of having to deny yourself something you forever crave.

33 - A Confidence Game of False Reassurances

Smoking is all about offering false reassurances. It promises pleasure but delivers only relief from the unpleasant withdrawal symptoms it itself causes. It promises concentration but only delivers relief from the distraction it itself causes. It promises relaxation but only delivers relief from the vexation it itself causes.

A confidence game is a swindle in which the victim is persuaded to trust the swindler in some way. Smokers come to believe that they need their cigarettes, that life without them is unimaginable, that life without cigarettes would be a protracted, desperate longing for cigarettes. Smokers rely on and trust cigarettes to provide them with various things of which smoking only provides illusions. The swindle rewards smokers by taking their health, their money, and by giving them the chains of addiction. You can have all this as long as you continue to smoke, but try to escape and you will be tormented for the rest of your days by your desire to smoke cigarettes.

Or so the story goes. What is not widely known is that it's not so difficult to cast off those chains if you understand the con game that's being played on you. Tobacco companies need and exploit *insecurity*. Insecurity that will accept false reassurances, that will accept illusion. When you are a teenager hovering around but not yet arrived into adulthood, you're insecure about being perceived as a child. You're desperate enough to be perceived as an adult that you just might do something ill-advised about it: start smoking to look like an adult. It's insecurity that starts people smoking, normally.

Another classic situation that starts slightly older people smoking is when they first enter the work force or, say, the military, and they are subject to a great deal of stress. Perhaps their colleagues or comrades smoke and tell them it helps deal with the stress and/or it seems like a way to fit in with the group. It's insecurity, again, that is exploited. Insecurity both about being able to handle the stress and also about fitting in with peers.

There's an important piece of writing titled Why and How the Tobacco Industry Sells Cigarettes to Young Adults: Evidence from Industry Documents by Pamela Ling and Stanton Glantz that depicts a tobacco industry that looks carefully into the available opportunities to exploit "uncertainty, stress and anxiety" in young adults; here is a quote in the Ling/Glance article from a 1984 document by people at a tobacco company:

> A young adult is leaving childhood on his way to adulthood. He is leaving the security and regiment of high school and his home. He is taking a new job; he is going to college; he is enlisting in the military. He is out on his own, with less support from his friends and family. These situations will be true for all generations of younger adults as they go through a period of transition from one world to another. . . . Dealing with these changes in his life will create increased levels of uncertainty, stress and anxiety. . . . During this stage in life, some younger adults will choose to smoke and will use smoking as a means of addressing some of these areas.[18]

Tobacco companies want to identify situations in which people are vulnerable to the false assurances they peddle so successfully. Get the young adults when they are uncertain, stressed, and anxious. Appeal to their insecurity.

But, of course, smoking doesn't help with stress. It just adds more stress. It adds many stresses: health concerns, financial concerns, and the stress of constant withdrawal symptoms. It's only when you smoke and experience relief from the withdrawal symptoms that the illusion of smoking as stress reducer seems viable. Ling and Glantz point this out. They say:

> Ironically, much of the stress that cigarettes relieve is caused by nicotine withdrawal; it is common for people who stop smoking, once they are past withdrawal, to feel less stress than they experienced while smoking. The use of smoking for "stress relief" as supported by tobacco marketing is really self-medication for nicotine withdrawal.[19]

Smoking has no real benefits, so it has to play forcefully to peoples' insecurities. It needs to offer reassurances to insecurities—false

18 See ncbi.nlm.nih.gov/pmc/articles/PMC1447481

19 Ibid.

reassurances—illusions of benefits—that, when accepted, come to seem like the real thing.

What the con artist *never* wants you to discover is *your own strength*, your own power. Because the con artist wants power over you, which requires that you put your trust in him/her, requires that you think you *need* him/her. Once you discover you don't need the con artist *at all*, the game is over. You are free of the dark illusions that have robbed you of your own power; you know the con artist has not been giving you the things you thought she/he was giving you. In the case of smoking, *you have supplied them yourself all along*.

Cigarettes don't reduce stress. They cause it. You yourself have been your stress reducer and manager. You have to give yourself credit for that because you deserve it. You've been managing stress all along, giving cigarettes credit they absolutely do not deserve. You can do it yourself, and the proof is that *you have been doing it yourself*. Not only have you been doing it yourself, but you've been doing it with the added stress of putting your trust in cigarettes, which have really only caused more stress.

34 - Other Smokers

Understanding how smokers react to those who stop smoking is important. Smokers often don't like it when other people stop smoking, particularly people with whom they smoke. It robs them of smoking companions. Another rat has left the ship, as Allen Carr puts it. It places smokers on the outside, again, isolates them on that ever-so-slowly sinking ship. Or out in that back alley, or wherever they have to go—away from everyone else—to feed the little monster. Also, with some, it can seem an implicit criticism of themselves that they have not stopped. When other people smoke with us, it validates our addiction.

Before I read Allen Carr's book, I stopped several times but relapsed in hanging out with friends who smoked. I'd go outside with them and not smoke but talk with them like we used to do when I smoked. That, in itself, was not a problem. But we'd also do a bit of drinking together, sometimes, and that was bad news. I'd eventually have a cigarette.

Smokers like company in their behavior. It helps justify their own behavior when others do it with them, especially in a convivial atmosphere. This is not evil behavior. It's understandable. Do not expect smokers to help you with any resolution about stopping smoking. A few may. But most would prefer to see you smoke like they do. So that they can smoke around you without discomfort and you support and justify their addiction by partaking in it also. Don't hate them for this. Understand it to be part of addiction.

When my mother was dying of cancer, one of my cousins came once a week to visit her. He was a heavy smoker. I had to ask him not to smoke in my mother's house. He stopped but he had to be asked. He would have continued had I not asked him not to smoke in the house.

My mother was a heavy smoker also. Until she became terminally ill with cancer. My parents' house had been smoker's paradise for decades.

When, some eight years previously, my father was dying of lung cancer, even I was smoking in the house. I have read the term 'addiction' defined as a behavior that the addict feels compelled to engage in even in the face of negative consequences. For themselves or others. I don't mean to paint them as uncaring monsters. To the contrary, my cousin was visiting because he did indeed care about my mother. And I loved my father deeply.

But addicts are caught in a web of lies and illusions that lead them to disregard their own health and welfare and that of others if and when it interferes in their feeding the addiction. Your stopping smoking is entirely up to you. Do not count on help from smokers.

Don't allow smoking in your dwelling, if possible. If there are friends who regularly smoke in it, set them up with a place to smoke outside, if possible. Supply a table, chairs, and an ashtray. If not possible, give them an ashtray. If they must smoke, they must do it outside.

If there are people who live with you who smoke inside, see if they are amenable to either smoking outside or only in one well-ventilated room if smoking outside is not feasible. You and others in the house are still exposed to it, of course, even if they limit their smoking to just one room, so it's best that they smoke outside.

There are good reasons to maintain your dwelling as smoke-free. Here are several reasons.

- It will be very encouraging and useful to you in your attempt to stop. Being exposed to smoke when you're trying to stop can be tempting.

- Tobacco smoke is highly toxic. When non-smokers enter a dwelling where someone smokes, they are not only revolted by the smell but also are concerned about their health.

- Especially if there are children in the house, non-smokers should not have to be both poisoned and revolted by smoke in the house. It is inconsiderate to expose others to such unpleasant toxicity.

- Smoking in a dwelling reduces the value of the dwelling.

- Keeping the smoking outside helps the smokers, also, in limiting their ability to smoke all the time.

And get rid of smoking materials in your dwelling, if possible, except an ashtray for your friends to smoke outside.

You don't have to join them outside when they smoke. You can if you want. They are used to smoking alone outside.

You need to take care of yourself. Be as accommodating to your friends as you can without allowing them to smoke inside your place or putting yourself in situations where you feel you are at risk of relapsing.

If friends don't understand this, they are not being good friends. Asking them to smoke outside is a reasonable request. Second-hand smoke causes cardiovascular disease, lung cancer, SIDS, and seriously harms children.[20] Even if you allowed smoking in your home previously, you and other non-smokers in the house, if there are others, should not have to suffer a toxic environment merely to convenience smokers who would prefer to smoke indoors.

If friends insists on smoking in your dwelling after you politely ask them not to, it's beyond rude; it's aggressive disregard of your well-being. Tell them to leave, if it is safe for you to do so.

If your partner or roommate refuses to smoke outside or in one and only one well-ventilated room, it will be especially important for you to dismantle your psychological addiction so that you are not especially tempted. And think about putting some distance between you and this person. It's one thing for smokers to smoke in places they shouldn't—before they are asked to desist. It's quite another for them to persist in it after they've been asked to stop. It shows no respect for you.

Most smokers, when asked to smoke outside, are not offended and agree to do that without argument or resentment. They know that smoking is toxic to non-smokers.

---

20 See

cdc.gov/tobacco/data_statistics/fact_sheets/secondhand_smoke/health
_effects

35 - The Truth and Other Smokers

A reason to stop smoking is to clear your mind of the web of lies and illusions that's part of being an addict. If you are a *lover of truth*—that is what the word *philosopher* means—then stopping smoking is also a means of attaining a little bit more mental clarity. When the smoke clears, you are better able to act with the compassion and good judgment you genuinely seek in your life—without having to be reminded what the appropriate action is by someone else.

Not to say that stopping smoking turns you into a wise person. Some ex-smokers lord their achievement over smokers in a way that infuriates smokers. Smokers are extremely sensitive around ex-smokers to judgment, be it moral, intellectual, or whatever.

An important part of being an ex-smoker is adopting progressive attitudes toward smokers. They need your help, but you need to remember some words of Friedrich Nietzsche, the German philosopher:

> Sometimes people don't want to hear the truth
> because they don't want their illusions destroyed.
> Friedrich Nietzsche from *Thus Spoke Zarathustra*

Destroying some illusions is crucial to dismantling the psychological dependence on smoking. But smokers who aren't ready to stop are not ready to hear the truth. They do indeed treasure their illusions about smoking and they do not want their illusions destroyed.

There is something pathetic about that, certainly. And they know it. But it doesn't help them to be ridiculed or tormented with their predicament. That doesn't help them stop smoking.

Allen Carr said the most important thing about his method is the way it *removes fear.* Smokers fear that if they quit, they'll experience great discomfort. Smoking, like other addictions, is self-medication to alleviate distress.

Con artists need the mark to experience fear. That's what keeps the mark from asking too many questions, that's what keeps them in line. That's what keeps them being marks. Smoking is a remote control con game. The tobacco companies don't need to send hoods in the night to extort the cash. They don't have to send anybody anytime.

They just need the addict to fear the idea of stopping smoking and to believe they need the poison to alleviate their distress and enjoy life.

It poisons the body but it also poisons the mind with fear and delusion. It poisons our ideas about enjoyment and pleasure. Cons have no regard for the health and welfare of the mark. They don't relent.

Smokers think that ex-smokers, particularly recent ones, feel envious of smokers smoking. Ex-smokers who haven't disabused themselves of the illusions of smoking do indeed suffer longings to smoke in the presence of smokers. But the way you're going about stopping smoking is to get rid of all desire for cigarettes. When you are in the presence of smokers smoking, you usually won't desire to smoke.

That will help the smokers realize it can be done without suffering a period of great torment. They will eventually be curious about how you managed to do it because they will see that you didn't suffer.

So you really don't need to say anything to them about your stopping smoking to help them. Remember that they are sensitive to losing fellow smokers. They would feel better if you had a smoke with them. But they don't need to feel bad just because you're not smoking, and they know that.

Your lack of discomfort will help them. It will help allay their fears that stopping smoking requires giving something up. But you have to keep quiet about it, unless they ask. Because "lectures" from ex-smokers is exactly what every smoker does not want. And, by the way, all you have to do is open your mouth about it and move your lips to make it a "lecture". Show the way by example until they explicitly ask about it.

You can help them. But remember that your having stopped, and *staying that way* is one of the biggest things you can do for *them* as well as for yourself. Showing the way by example is going to work much better than many words. And as they see you with a new enjoyment and involvement in life, with a renewed sense of enjoyment and pleasure, they'll of course notice and eventually be curious. It's likely that they too want to stop smoking: "Among all current U.S. adult cigarette smokers, nearly 7 out of every 10 (68.8%) reported in 2010 that they wanted to quit completely".[21]

---

21 cdc.gov/tobacco/data_statistics/fact_sheets/cessation/quitting

36 - Compassion Toward Other Smokers

Dr Gabor Maté and A. H. Almass note that "Only when compassion is present will people allow themselves to see the truth." You can't help smokers stop without feeling compassion toward them.

People don't want their illusions destroyed, because they're comforting. They'll only be willing to entertain the possibility that their pet illusion is indeed an illusion in the presence of a compassion that neither beats them with the truth nor sees them as stupid for not recognizing it as an illusion.

Their illusion not only comforts them but is medication against discomfort. Depriving someone of their pet illusion deprives them of their medication against psychological distress. If you deprive someone of their meds, they want a sense that it's in their best interest and they will not be left without something to alleviate the distress the medication was for. They need to sense you understand and sympathize with them on this.

The illusion is that smoking alleviates distress other than the distress it itself causes via withdrawal symptoms. The replacement for the 'medication' provided by smoking includes realizing that not only is smoking bad medicine indeed—it *creates* more distress than it alleviates—but smokers have been dealing with their distress themselves, all this time—it's been they themselves who have alleviated their distress, not the smoking.

They'll also need to look at why they've continued to smoke. What is so distressing that they've continued to poison themselves with this addiction for years? What is so distressing that this deadly 'medication' is preferable to stopping?

To find out, they need to be able to not deny or avoid their own psychological pain, but just be with it, feel it, check it out. Avoiding and denying pain causes more pain than simply being there and feeling it. Dealing with things, whether it's psychological pain, or the bills, or other responsibilities, is the only way the situation improves. And it isn't so bad, once you get started. Avoiding it is the most painful part.

37 - Once an Addict Always an Addict?

Allen Carr says the old maxim "Once an addict, always an addict" is not true. Alcoholics Anonymous says it's true. Which is it?

Carr says he respects AA because it doesn't exploit addicts; it helps them. I agree and also respect AA for that reason. Carr says his method is a full cure of nicotine addiction, so that people cured by his method are not addicts anymore; while he respects AA, he differs with them on the issue of "Once an addict, always an addict".

I respect AA and Carr, but I don't agree with either of them on the issue of "Once and addict, always an addict". In short, when you stop smoking, you won't be an addict but you won't be as safe from it as someone who never smoked.

As George Carlin put it, "Just cuz you got the monkey off your back doesn't mean the circus has left town." You won't have to fight an ongoing, torturous battle of willpower to keep yourself from smoking, but there will be times, which grow more infrequent over time, when you will have to deal with some sort of desire for cigarettes.

Smokers sometimes don't try to stop because they think they will continue to want cigarettes the rest of their lives and will have to exercise immense willpower once they stop. In short, they think "once an addict, always an addict".

It's not true that you will have to fight an excruciating, ongoing battle of willpower over urges to smoke. You can get rid of your desire for cigarettes.

But what does that mean? It means that you are dismantling the psychological addiction to smoking and, after a week of no smoking, will have ditched the physical addiction. It means that you ditch almost all of the desire to smoke early on—not just the physical addiction but the urge to smoke also. But there can be parts of it that remain that you get out of your system over a longer time. It doesn't involve the excruciating, ongoing battle that occurs when continual urges are involved. There will be skirmishes, though. But even if urges happen occasionally, you have the tools to deal with them.

A psychological addiction to smoking is, in large part, an attitude to smoking. You like them. You gotta have em. You think they're great. You think they taste great. You think they relax you. You think you almost go to heaven when you have one. You keen for the smell of them before they're lit. On and on. You can get all of this out of your head and out of your heart. But it isn't like a disease where, once healed, that's it, you don't have it any more. You can assume an attitude briefly that you once had but don't really have anymore. Like you can remember what you felt for someone you don't love anymore. But that doesn't mean that just because you can remember, you have to fall in love with them again.

Some people do indeed never desire a cigarette ever again. But it also seems common to experience an initial period in which there are no urges for cigarettes, just the mild hunger and light-headedness of the little monster for a week, which is actually easier to deal with than hunger for food, as long as the amplifier is dismantled and you aren't experiencing urges. Then, eventually, many people experience what might be likened to occasional, mild involuntary twitches of desire for a cigarette. Like the little monster is rolling over in its grave. Not urges, not very strong, but something like a mild involuntary twitch of desire.

I still find it interesting to watch some smokers smoke, sometimes. Not because I envy them, but because sometimes they're expressive. Usually it doesn't make me want to smoke, myself. Sometimes it does, though, briefly. Not strongly. Like a twitch. A pale shadow of the former 'urges'. But there it is. I proceed with caution, in that event. Probably it also has to do with the fact that my mother smoked a lot when I was a child; I didn't like the smell of it—it felt like an assault on me—but I like the look of it, sometimes, going back, no doubt, to my early youth.

Long ago I fell out of love with smoking—the romance is over, for me —and fell in love with a different life without smoking. I am clear that smoking does not provide me any of the things I thought it did, when I smoked. But it wouldn't take much for me to be smoking again.

I don't have to deal with the urges I had to deal with before I read Allen Carr's book. But I am not a rational creature all the time. Sometimes I just want one. However, at those times, I am in a better position to deal with it. I am not a Buddhist, but there is great value in what they have to say about observing your emotions and desires. It's possible to observe them with some detachment. So that they do not carry you away. And they drift away like smoke.

It does not pay to think you are above the power of tobacco to enslave you, whether you have never smoked a cigarette in your life or have smoked for thirty years. That is a kind of hubris, or tragic pride, that does not end well. You think you are above it so you find out the hard way you aren't. The word 'hubris' goes back to ancient Greece; it's a very old story.

For instance, in *The Bacchae*, an ancient tragedy by Euripides (about 2300 years old), Dionysus, the god of wine and revelry, comes to town (Thebes). King Pentheus displays hubris toward Dionysus. Pentheus doesn't have respect for Dionysus or his powers. To Pentheus, Dionysus is about wanton abandon, drunkenness, and disrespect for civil order—which Pentheus controls. It doesn't end at all well for King Pentheus. First, Dionysus dominates him, controls him. Dionysus suggests to Pentheus that he should dress up like a woman to spy on the women of the city, including Pentheus's mother, who have traveled to the woods outside the city and are reportedly behaving unseemly there as revelers and followers of Dionysus. Pentheus doesn't like it and wants to send in troops to kill some of them and bring them back to the city. Dionysus convinces Pentheus it would be better to first spy on them dressed up as a woman. So Pentheus, befuddled, dresses up as a woman and spies on the women. Dionysus points him out to the female revelers, including Pentheus's mother, who mistake him for a mountain lion and tear him limb from limb.

You probably don't need to worry about being torn limb from limb by a ferocious bunch of female followers of Dionysus (Maenads). But the point is that just as alcohol, as a psychoactive addictive substance, can dominate people and their lives—seemingly like a god from on-high—so too can tobacco and smoking.

Tobacco and nicotine are powerful and can dominate peoples' will, as we know. People have known and revered tobacco and its power for thousands of years. If you want to be free of domination by tobacco, it does not pay to think you are above being dominated by it. That is tragic pride and you could pay by being dominated once again by it.

Because if you think you are above being dominated by it, you might think you can smoke one here or there and you won't go back to smoking. But of course there simply is no such thing as 'only one'. *You are hooked when you want a cigarette*; the addiction is primarily psychological. You are simply landed when you smoke one. You must acknowledge the power of tobacco to dominate your will if you are going to avoid fooling yourself into thinking you can have one without going back to smoking regularly.

There are many ways to fool yourself into smoking a cigarette, once you stop. If you're Jonesing for a smoke, almost any of them seem convincing. But if you're not seriously Jonesing for a smoke, they don't look so good, and they're not so convincing. They're sometimes funny. In any case, if you're Jonesing, the romance is not over, for you, with smoking. Jonesing is pining for a cigarette like an adolescent pines for his girlfriend. Or like a puppy whimpers for its owner.

The cure of smoking that you are working on right now can indeed be permanent and indeed be a total cure in that you no longer desire to smoke. If you don't smoke and you no longer desire to smoke, you're a non-smoker and you aren't a nicotine addict.

38 - The Pleasure of Breathing and the Pleasure of Smoking

A friend whom I am currently helping stop smoking doesn't believe that there is no real pleasure in smoking. She describes it as a "guilty pleasure".

> i do feel guilty every time i pick one up but i do so enjoy it.. i guess that's what they mean by guilty pleasure. Though for what it's worth, your words resonate with me EVERY SINGLE time i even think about picking one up -- but there's a teenage rebellious girl in me who wants to be "bad" -- to beat the system... a weird thrill in doing what i know im not supposed to.

I recall that sort of 'pleasure' in smoking. That is part of what I refer to as the *romance* with smoking. This particular part of the romance is the pleasure of being bad, being transgressive, of crossing the line from obedience into rebellion. Of course there's also a sexual dimension to it. I remember basically lusting for a cigarette.

To the smoker caught in this tangle of desires, the idea that one can extricate oneself from it may seem like the idea that one can change one's sexual preference—*forget it*. But it isn't that way, actually. It's more like extracting yourself emotionally from an abusive relationship. It may take a bit of time and a bit of reflection, but it is eminently doable—and even inevitable once you have read this book and your perspective is changed on smoking and stopping smoking. First your mind changes. Then your heart catches up.

We've talked about this earlier in the book, but it's worth exploring more. I think it's important to develop an appreciation of the pleasure of breathing. It may seem like something that is without pleasure. But all that means is you have no appreciation for it, yet. Because, if we learn one thing from smoking, it's that even the most toxic, foul, revolting, addictive poison can be found pleasurable if only we think it so and persist in it.

Which brings us to the nature of pleasure. What is pleasurable? Some people think that real pleasure is derived from what is *natural*, in some sense, and that everything else is not really pleasurable.

But I think it's quite clear that, on the contrary, we can have a big role in deciding what we find pleasurable and in developing our own tastes. If we have an interest in culture, we can develop our tastes in a wide variety of directions.

We can develop—and change—our own tastes in a similar way to how we develop and change our own sense of the meaning of life.

What is the meaning of life? Some would say there is an absolute way it is and we merely *discover* what it is. But I think we *create* our own meaning via a process of both *discovery* and *creation*. When we interpret the meaning of language, we interpret the meaning of something that is *ambiguous*. It could mean various things. We select one. We choose. That's what it means to create meaning. There often is no absolute right choice. We discover and invent in a long series of discoveries and choices that add up to a big interpretation that may be uniquely ours. Just like if everyone chooses a number between 1 and 999,999,999,999,999,999,999,999,999,999,999,999,999,999,999,999,999,999,999, everyone is likely to pick a different number than everyone else because there are so many possibilities to choose among.

What we find pleasurable is not absolute, either. There probably isn't anything that *everyone* finds pleasurable. Sex? There are many who don't enjoy it. Chocolate? Believe it or not, there are those who don't like it. Why is there nothing universally pleasurable? Because while our biological chemistry and our psychological needs predispose us in certain directions, what we find pleasurable is like what we find the meaning of life to be: it's *discovered and created by us* over time through a long series of experiences and choices that form our tastes. It's a mental construct, not simply something that is biologically determined.

So we ourselves are the ones who decide what the meaning of life is, to some extent, and we also decide what we find pleasurable, to some extent. And these things can change slowly over time as we move in new directions.

The point is that once you change your perspective on smoking and stopping smoking by reading this book, you start to question what you get from smoking. You start to realize that it doesn't give you what you thought it was giving you. Eventually you will realize that the 'pleasure of smoking' is a mental construct rather than something that is biologically determined by the mixture of our chemistry with the chemistry of tobacco. And you will tear that construct apart, dismantling your psychological addiction by dispelling the illusions it depends on.

In the meantime, one thing that will help you a lot with the transition from being a smoker to being a non-smoker is cultivating an appreciation for the pleasure of breathing. It may seem like a simple thing that holds no pleasure. But it can easily be appreciated for the pleasures and, really, the wonders it holds, properly understood.

Let's compare and contrast it with the 'pleasures' of smoking.

Smoking is inseparably an act of breathing. But it's poisonous. Whereas breathing fresh air is the opposite of poisonous. It's an infusion of life-force, of prana, of sustaining energy, of crucial oxygen, rather than a hit of a drug that slowly robs you of your health.

So of course breathing is not a "guilty pleasure". There's no guilt. It's pleasure without guilt. Not only is there no guilt, but there's even a sense of achievement and growth in coming to an appreciation of the pleasures of breathing.

With each drag of a cigarette, you pay a rotten company for a rotten product that represents some of the worst that corporate capitalism has to offer. Breathing fresh air—if you can find it—is free.

To experience the pleasure of breathing, you don't need to carry any packages. No lighter. No ashtray. No cigarettes. You just breathe slowly and deeply. It's convenient. All the gear you need comes fully supplied with a human body.

All wound up? Take a deep breath. Actually, take twenty. Then relax. Then do it again. Guaranteed to make you feel better. More relaxed. Works better than smoking. Smoking gives you relief from withdrawal symptoms. But it makes your heart rate increase. It simply gets rid of the distracting withdrawal symptoms. Smoking makes you feel like a normal person, temporarily, by getting rid of withdrawal symptoms. Whereas slow, deep breathing makes everyone feel more relaxed.

Need to concentrate? The only help smoking gives you is relief from withdrawal symptoms. So that you are better able to concentrate. Whereas deep breathing is the very root of inspiration. *Inspiration* means to breathe in.

Learning to breathe through your nose is very good. It makes for less phlegm in your throat that is very hard to move. Because breathing though your mouth, particularly at night when you're sleeping, creates that phlegm. Breathing through your nose is much preferable to breathing through your mouth. The Buteyko Breathing Technique proposes the use of breathing exercises as a treatment for asthma as well as other conditions. It helps you learn how to breathe through your nose while you're sleeping—and the rest of the time.

The pleasure, for non-smokers, of breathing through your nose has several components. First, there are all the health benefits of breathing through your nose. If you have asthma, breathing through your nose can help you a great deal. If you experience snoring or sleep apnea, learning to breathe through your nose when sleeping helps you with those problems. Air intake is slightly slower through the nose than through the mouth, and that slowness is better suited to the amount of air we need.

Secondly, since our sense of smell is in the nose, breathing through your nose most or all of the time provides a life experience more attuned to the smells around you. This is a more sensual experience.

Thirdly, when you breathe through your nose, you can feel the temperature of the air. You feel the coolness in your nostrils. You feel the air more.

Whether you breathe through your nose or through your mouth, there are other pleasures associated with breathing.

When you take a deep breath, you feel the muscles in your rib cage stretch a bit. This stretching feels good. It always feels like the more we stretch those muscles, the greater the air capacity of our lungs can be. It feels good the same way stretching your muscles feels when you're tired and you stretch your body.

I jog and exercise. To help me do the work, I look for the pleasure of breathing. I consciously enjoy the top of a breath, when my lungs are full. I consciously enjoy the rhythm of the breathing, the percussion. Being sensitive to the pleasure of breathing helps you get more enjoyment out of exercise which, in turn, helps you do it regularly.

There's also the pleasure of knowing that, in your breathing practice and exercises, you have a tool at your disposal which is better than smoking at helping you with stress, worry, and concentration. And this is a tool that isn't an addictive drug that hurts you more than it helps you. This tool helps you move your very spirit in positive directions. The word *spirit* means *breath*. How you feel has a lot to do with how you breath. And how you breath influences how you feel. Taking conscious control of your breathing helps you take control of yourself and your life, whereas smoking puts you under the remote control of a tobacco company.

Cultivating an appreciation for the pleasures of breathing helps you in many ways. Not only does it contribute to your health and well-being by giving you the health and psychological benefits we've discussed, but it also makes you value being able to breathe without smoking. Smoking impairs your breathing. It decreases your lung capacity, it makes you wheeze, it impairs your sense of smell and just generally makes breathing a lot less enjoyable. Appreciating the pleasures of breathing helps you stay away from smoking to enjoy the pleasures and benefits of breathing.

Cultivating an appreciation for the pleasures of breathing can be an interesting, ongoing thing in your life. Like the cultivation of taste and pleasure in the arts, for instance. That isn't a process that stops. One keeps on learning and appreciating both old and new things one has seen and learned.

The very simple act of breathing, it turns out, has profound depths that are ours to explore, contemplate, enjoy, and benefit from.

39 - Checklist If You Want to Smoke

If you are comfortable with the idea that smoking doesn't give you what you thought it gave you but, instead, offers only empty illusions of benefits, then your 'urges' to smoke are either gone or are sufficiently diminished that the word 'twinges' is more descriptive, now, of how you feel. Although you may sometimes experience twinges, they will not be the sort of strong urges that kept you smoking previously. You will have dismantled the amplifier, so you won't experience 'urges'. Or even if you do, you can turn off the amplifier and take the screwdriver to it again. You are learning how to deal with your addiction, dismantle it, observe yourself, and be in touch with yourself to know if you still desire to smoke. If you do, try these things.

- Take as many deep, easy breaths as it takes for you to feel better. Feel the pleasure of breathing fresh air. Feel the energizing effect of your breathing. Research breathing exercises on the Internet. Find ones you like for different situations. Kundalini yoga's pranayama is very useful. Learn how to use breathing exercises to help with stress reduction, concentration, and *life force.*

- Consider the situations, places, times and moods in which you previously would smoke. Anticipate these 'trigger situations' and plan to minimize the occurrence of those situations or plan on how you will deal with them when they arise. Substitutes are OK if you are still feeling urges. For instance, if you reward yourself in some situations with a cigarette, plan a different healthier, more interesting reward. If you smoke when you're nervous, work out some breathing exercises that work better than smoking. If you smoke to concentrate, work out some breathing exercises that work better than smoking.

- Appreciate your freedom from the dependence of addiction; summon your joy and gratitude for being free from it.

- Consider why you continued to smoke and that it does not give you any of the things you thought it did. Eventually the desire to smoke is as powerless over you as the magic of a card trick you understand.

- Look at your twinge for a cigarette. What is it really a desire for? What is that desire masking? What sort of distress is it in response to? Deal with the distress differently than by smoking.

- Acknowledge the power of tobacco to dominate you. Realize you have to keep your distance.

- Know that the twinge is momentary and will disappear like a wisp of smoke. And, over time, these twinges will happen less and less until you have no desire at all to smoke.

- Observe your desire to smoke as though from a distance, with some detachment. Not as though it was happening to someone else (don't be numb to it), but as though you can see it happening to yourself, as though you can see yourself from a slight distance. Just feel it, observe it, and let it pass.

Once the physical addiction is over, which takes about a week, any desire you have to smoke is purely psychological. But of course the addiction is 99% psychological. Once the physical addiction is over, you are dealing solely with the psychological dependence.

There's the desire for a cigarette, and there's the distress (or something else) the cigarette is meant to medicate or accompany. What is that distress or other feeling about? Don't be afraid to feel that distress/other feeling. You can feel it without being engulfed by it. What is the cause of it? How to deal with it apart from smoking?

As time goes on, you will begin to see your nicotine addiction's mechanisms ever more clearly, like a pile of dismantled machinery that occasionally needs some inspection and tinkering to keep it dismantled. Those occasional little twinges won't be excruciating or torturous. The urges are or will be pretty much gone. But those twinges will tell you where the machinery of your addiction needs a screwdriver to keep it dismantled.

So is it true that once you are an addict you will always be an addict? Well, no. But it pays to acknowledge and respect the power of tobacco to dominate your will. If you are willing to fool yourself into thinking it can't or won't dominate your will, you've got misplaced confidence that will deliver you into servitude. Not because you are still an addict. But because that's how smoking creates addicts and keeps them being addicts.

It's all about desire and illusion. The ex-smoker who has a cigarette doesn't think he's going to be smoking regularly soon any more than the gambling addict thinks he isn't going to recoup his losses in the next round. It's about desire and illusion, being willing to fool yourself and insist on the reality of a fantasy.

40 - I'll Just Have One and Only One

Previous to reading Allen Carr's book, whenever I quit and then eventually broke down and had one, that was it. Game over. I never managed to just have one and only one. Or if I did, it wasn't for long; eventually I had another and was soon back at it regularly.

There is almost never any such thing as *one and only one*, with smoking. As soon as you want it you're hooked like a fish. Smoking the cigarette is when you're landed. The main illusion involved in cigarette addiction is that you enjoy it. As soon as that illusion is fully operational, you're hooked, whether you are smoking or not. Given how displeasurable, noxious, filthy, disgusting, and foul tasting cigarettes truly are, the illusion that you enjoy them is not a simple one to sustain. If you think you enjoy them, you're going to want one. And if you want one, you're eventually going to have one. And if you eventually have one, you're eventually going to have two. And so on.

If you know you don't enjoy smoking but you have one all the same, again, you're already hooked. Even if you have it to confirm that you're not hooked. One of the infuriating, mystifying things about smoking is that you can stop smoking, know you don't enjoy smoking, not even really want one and somehow end up smoking a cigarette all the same, loathing the taste and experience of it but hooked again all the same. How does that happen?

For some people, it's because they haven't fully understood why they continue to smoke. Perhaps they understand that they don't enjoy it and that smoking doesn't help them concentrate or relax or help them manage stress. But perhaps there are additional reasons. Some people smoke when they get depressed and/or don't feel good about themselves. I've done that. I just didn't care anymore. About me or anything else. Smoking a cigarette was an act of self-destruction and also flipping the bird to the world. It was an act of surrender to the feeling that I deserve lousy things in my life like being a slave to smoking.

They say that depression is rage turned inward. So it seems with me. Partly at myself. Partly at others. Partly just in general. But here's something that may help you avoid smoking in those situations if you are vulnerable there. If you relapse into smoking, you don't just hurt yourself. You help a whole disgusting industry with their corporate revenue. You help the tobacco company whose cigarettes you're buying. They happily would sell you poison till you kill yourself with it. They'll sell it to you and millions of other people, as many as possible. And, what's more, they know that people experiencing depression are great customers and they probably go after them with all the enthusiasm of jackals for a wounded animal. So put that rage to good use. Don't help tobacco companies. Don't hurt them, but don't help them, either. They're counting on you to buy their poison. They think they own you. They think you're weak and they think they know exactly how to exploit that weakness. Don't help them.

41 - Mental Illness and Smoking

Many people suffering from mental illness smoke. But stopping smoking is better for your mental health than smoking. It's good for your mental health to stop smoking for a variety of reasons. Dr. Lion Shahab of University College London says, in the British Journal of Psychiatry:

> Stopping smoking is the single most important step anyone can take to improve their health, whatever their age. Our findings show that quitting does not worsen and, if anything improves mental health, even after life-long smoking. However, smokers with depression may require more help so clinicians should support cessation to reduce health inequalities. [22]

First of all, stopping smoking improves your mental health because it's so very consequential in improving your physical health. You feel better in so many ways. Your circulation is better so you aren't as tired. You don't wheeze anymore so you don't feel so sick. You feel stronger, more energetic. You can smell more acutely. You're better in the sack because circulation is so important to the proper functioning of sex organs. You actually feel like getting some exercise. These dramatic improvements in physical health make you feel better mentally.

Secondly, when you realize that smoking does not provide you with the health or other benefits that you thought it did, and that you have been providing those benefits to yourself all this time, and that rather than helping you, smoking has in fact been hurting you all this time, your mental health improves. This is an empowering realization. You realize that not only do you not need to smoke, but that stopping smoking will not rob you of anything you enjoy or value. You realize that stopping smoking gets rid of a blood sucking parasite that has

---

22 Dr. Lion Shahab, British Journal of Psychiatry, May 2015, "Reciprocal associations between smoking cessation and depression in older smokers: findings from the English Longitudinal Study of Ageing", http://bjp.rcpsych.org/content/early/2015/05/11/bjp.bp.114.153494 . See also a review of this research at http://www.rcpsych.ac.uk/mediacentre/pressreleases2015/olderpeople andsmoking.aspx

been supping on your health, pocket book—and mental health—for years. Stopping smoking is good for your mental health because you realize that smoking is more of a contributor to stress, anxiety, fear and depression than it is an aide against these things.

Stopping smoking is good for your mental health because it makes you laugh. You see how strong illusions can be in shaping our behavior and you rid yourself of some of them. The illusions that you enjoyed smoking, that it helped you, that you needed it, that it's hard to stop—all these illusions were unshakable realities yesterday. Finding the truth is exciting, empowering, and good for your mental health.

Stopping smoking is good for your mental health because, done properly, it's an exciting revelation of the truth. It's freeing. Stopping smoking is good for your mental health because it's an experience of gaining freedom from a kind of servitude. It feels great in every possible way, and you don't have to give up anything that you truly enjoy or value.

Moreover, Shahab's research indicates that even those who are life-long smokers who suffer from depression do not experience any increased depression from stopping smoking.

But what all this does not mean is that stopping smoking cures clinical depression or that all 'medicine' does not work. Stopping smoking will be good for the mental health of those who are clinically depressed for the above reasons, but it won't necessarily cure their clinical depression. One thing at a time. Stop smoking. That will be a big help. Get medical help with depression, if you are seriously depressed. Stopping smoking may be, as Dr. Shahab says, "the single most important thing anyone can do to improve their health", but for those who are seriously depressed, getting some help with depression is at least equally important.

42 - Will I Gain Weight?

It's commonly held that you gain weight when you stop smoking. If you substitute eating for smoking, then you gain weight. But it's not inevitable that you must substitute eating for smoking. The way we're going about it does not involve substitutions. You don't need them. If you don't desire a cigarette, you don't need a substitute. *You don't need a substitute for something you don't want.*

You will probably experience *less* hunger when you stop smoking. Here's why. Smokers are constantly in various stages of nicotine withdrawal. It's a kind of hunger for nicotine. But when you stop smoking, it's only a matter of a few days before that physical hunger for nicotine disappears. When you stop smoking you get rid of a hunger imposed on you by an addiction.

Many of the indigenous peoples of the Americas believe/d that tobacco is/was the food of the Spirits, and thought of the physical sensation of nicotine withdrawal as the hunger of the spirits for their food: tobacco. So that humans experienced both their own hunger for their own food and, if they were smokers/snuff chewers/etc, the additional hunger of the spirits for their own different type of food. Getting rid of one type of hunger makes for a lot less hunger.

When I was a smoker, I remember experiencing nicotine withdrawal sometimes as a hunger that I tried to satisfy by eating. In any case, you won't experience that sort of hunger any more.

Some smokers find smoking helps them as a hunger suppressant, helps them not need to eat very much. This is not a universal experience among smokers, however; others find that they experience more hunger as a smoker. That was my case, as I've said. However, those who have used smoking as a hunger suppressant will have to amp up the exercise.

After you stop smoking, you begin to find the idea of exercise appealing. I didn't exercise when I smoked. I wheezed and had a terrible smoker's cough. The idea of exercising was out of the question. My body was under stress from smoking.

After I stopped, I slowly started to get into exercising. Over the years, I've lost 45 pounds and increased the amount of exercise from a 20 minute walk to a 4-10km jog several times per week. I'm in my fifties and feel better now than I did in my thirties and forties.

When you stop smoking, very soon you aren't wheezing and coughing anymore. Your lung capacity increases. Your blood circulation improves. This gives you more energy in all sorts of departments including sexual energy.

When you stop smoking, you soon find yourself with a more energetic body than when you smoked. This newly energized body and you should get to know one another. Take it for walks. Give it some exercise. You will find a new joy in exercising. It gets rid of aches and pains. And it makes you feel good. Makes you feel alive.

Figure out ways to enjoy and exercise what will soon be your newly energetic body. Everybody past their 30's has to exercise or they gain weight. Make exercise a part of your life regularly. It makes you feel much better. And it helps keep your weight down.

Smoking increases your metabolic rate—your body burns energy faster. So that's another reason to start exercising or amp it up if you already are exercising. Stopping smoking decreases your metabolic rate and so does aging. Exercise combats that decrease in metabolic rate very effectively. When your metabolic rate decreases, you gain weight if you eat the same amount of food as before—unless you exercise to make up for those calories you're not burning otherwise.

Your metabolic rate is going to decrease as you age whether you stop smoking or not. Smokers and non-smokers alike gain weight as they get older unless they rethink their diet and exercise. You're going to have to deal with it whether you stop smoking or not. You deal with it mainly by diet and exercise.

And by stopping smoking. Smoking makes you sedentary. No one wants to exercise when they wheeze like an old set of bagpipes. But when you stop smoking, you can look forward to rediscovering or discovering that you have a body. A body that enjoys being taken out for walkies exactly as much dogs like being taken for walkies. It's a really exciting part of stopping smoking to get physical again. And if you do, you won't gain weight.

And get those new lungs pumping good air through your body. Learn what breathing exercises feel good to you and help you with stress, relaxation, concentration, and general health. Take some deep breaths and feel suffused with life.

43 - Stopping Smoking is an Exciting Experience

There's a lot of misinformation about stopping smoking. It's described as a terrible experience. It's not true that it's necessarily a bad experience. There is more physical discomfort when you stop drinking coffee than when you stop smoking. Stopping smoking should be known as a fantastic experience. Because you get over some illusions that weigh like albatrosses around your neck. You discard some illusions that profit blood-suckers supping on you. And you see that illusions are more powerful than you thought they could be.

With drugs like LSD, the attraction is the hallucination, the exquisite illusion and, in general, drugs are known for the illusions they create. But the whole mechanism of addiction is about illusion and desire. The whole illusion that you want and need the drug is the main thing to understand about drugs and their illusions. You don't need it. The urges for it are mostly amplified desire for the things you think it gives you. That is what you are desperate for; not the drug. Once you fully understand that smoking doesn't give you any of the things you think it gives you, the urges disappear. Gone. Never to return. Vanished like smoke. The illusion is over. And you are free. When you understand a 'magic' trick, you are not subject to the illusion any more. The same is true of smoking.

Stopping smoking is the best smoking-related experience you can have. And if you read this book and Allen Carr's book, you can have it the way it should be done: without having to exercise unmanageable levels of willpower. That's exciting.

44 - Cigarettes and Enjoyment

Cigarettes provide relief from the nicotine withdrawal symptoms that they themselves create. That is what the "enjoyment" of cigarettes mainly is: temporary relief from the discomfort that cigarettes create.

If someone were to follow you around and regularly poke you in the ribs until you took one of the cancerous poison pills they sold you regularly, you wouldn't say you enjoy the pills. You simply feel relief from being extorted.

To confuse enjoyment with relief is to let an appreciation of real enjoyment be stolen from you. Cigarettes steal your ability to appreciate real enjoyment. Even while smokers think they couldn't really enjoy life without cigarettes.

What sort of enjoyment can come from scratching an itch when scratching the itch is what causes more itching in the future? We all know that one, smokers and non-smokers alike. We scratch it even though we know it's going to cause more itching. Because the temporary relief from the itch seems heavenly, seems enjoyable.

But we wouldn't confuse it with enjoyment. Confusing enjoyment with relief from suffering is not exactly masochistic, which involves an 'enjoyment' of suffering itself (as opposed to 'enjoying' the relief of suffering, in the case of smokers), but it's related. Particularly when relieving the suffering simply sets up and guarantees more suffering in the future. Which is how addictions work. Both involve a degraded version of 'enjoyment'. 'Enjoyment' has the word 'joy' in it. 'Enjoyment' of cigarettes is joyless. Relief from the irritation of withdrawal symptoms is different from experiencing joy. They aren't mutually exclusive, but they shouldn't be confused with one another.

When we get a *real* itch that won't go away, we get rid of the itch with creams or pills or whatever, normally. But getting rid of the itch for cigarettes is a bit different. Because the itch is 99% psychological. There is a physical component, but it's relatively insignificant compared to the dramatic nature of cravings for cigarettes. Cravings are primarily psychological rather than simply physical though, of course, to smokers they seem extremely and utterly physical.

It's much easier to ditch cigarettes when you understand that *you never really enjoyed them in the first place*. That is one of the main illusions that needs to be debunked so that you can see that cigarettes do not really give you any of the good things you think they give you. Including enjoyment.

When you have a cigarette and experience relief from the discomfort of withdrawal symptoms, it isn't so much that you feel pleasure or enjoyment; you simply no longer feel the discomfort of the withdrawal symptoms. In short, you temporarily feel like a non-smoker. Smokers smoke to rid themselves of the irritation of withdrawal symptoms. They smoke to temporarily feel like non-smokers.

The good news is that when this and a few other key illusions about smoking are fully dismantled in your own mind, smoking no longer has a hold on you. You don't feel the cravings any more. They're gone. Permanently. And how easy would it be to stop smoking if you no longer wanted to smoke? It's easy, then. That is why Allen Carr calls it "The Easy Way to Stop Smoking". It doesn't require a lot of willpower. How much willpower would be required if you didn't want to smoke?

That's like asking how much willpower would be required to not cross the road if you didn't want to cross the road. Not much. How much willpower would be required not to scratch a wound if it didn't itch? Not much. The key is to get rid of the itch. So that you don't need unreasonable amounts of willpower.

45 - The Importance & Pleasure of Being Bad

We've talked about "the pleasures of smoking" being illusory. It promises pleasure but delivers only relief from torment it itself exacts, and the relief makes future torment inevitable. Smoking establishes an unfair settlement. We settle not for real pleasure but for relief from the torments of withdrawal symptoms. But are there other less illusory "pleasures" associated with smoking?

It's important to think about the pleasure of being bad. It isn't the pleasure of stabbing someone in the face. That's being very bad indeed, but there is no pleasure in it for anybody in their right mind. The pleasure of being bad is the pleasure of disobeying a rule, law or convention that *should* be disobeyed. As when protesters engage in civil disobedience to protest unjust laws. Or when graffiti artists create 'the writing on the wall' that is illegal but provides an important message that isn't seen elsewhere. Or when young people defy dowdy rules of dress in in celebration of individuality, flamboyancy, and sexuality. Or when artists/inventors create something original contrary to the previous 'rules of the game'.

The pleasure of being bad is the pleasure of defying authority, tradition/expectation, and the forces of dullness. The pleasure of being bad is the pleasure of feeling alive.

The pleasure of being bad is too important to confuse it with smoking. To smoke is to be enslaved to the forces of dullness. You pay lots of money to people who sell poison as something that helps people and gives them pleasure but in fact does neither. To smoke is not to be a rebel for individuality, justice or anything admirable. It's to be a dupe of big corporations. It's to trust the wrong people. It's to be a victim of one's own insecurities. It's to have been taken in by a confidence game played by unscrupulous, uncaring companies.

To smoke is not to be bad, in the good sense of being bad. It's important to reclaim the notion of what it means to be bad. Because when people associate the idea of being daring and a rebel with smoking, they are settling for a degraded version of those important notions. They are settling for pathetic and slow self-destruction concerning what it means to be a rebel when, instead, the real rebels are very far indeed from pathetic and self-destructive.

46 - Being Around Smokers and Alcohol

After you stop smoking, how do you deal with your friends and associates who smoke? Carefully. You deal with them carefully. Keep in mind that though they may love you, if they smoke, they may prefer to see you smoking. It's one of the impairments of judgment that often accompanies smoking. It doesn't make them monsters. They smoke, so they view it as a given that other people should smoke. Keep it in mind.

So you would be well advised not to drink around them at least for several months. When people drink, their judgment is impaired. They do things they don't do when sober. I mean you. Several of my early attempts to stop smoking were scuttled when I drank alcohol. And then had a cigarette. There is almost never such a thing as one and only one cigarette. I had to learn this the hard way as do many.

I eventually concluded that if I was going to stop smoking, I would have to stop drinking also. But, then, drinking was a problem for me. It caused me problems. I would open my mouth and what came out would, too often, be a problem. Sometimes I would say hurtful things that I *didn't even believe*. My judgment and my character were sometimes altered for the worse when I drank. I was a worse person when I drank, sometimes.

Was I an alcoholic? I don't know. But I had a drinking problem. When I'd drink, I was a problem. Mainly for me, but also for friends and colleagues, sometimes.

Also, when I was trying to stop smoking, my weight was high. I wasn't exercising. And the alcohol was helping put more pounds on me. I was smoking, drinking, overweight and out of shape. I was starting to ache all the time. Back problems. Gravity. Headaches. In my forties.

First I quit drinking. That was easier for me than stopping smoking. Stopping drinking wasn't that hard for me. When I drink I'm not very good at what I like to do, which is write and program computers to do arty things. Also, I am not as much of an asshole when I'm not drinking. Alcohol was not giving me anything anymore, if it ever did. It was just turning me into an overweight big mouth.

Once I'd successfully stopped drinking, I tried stopping smoking via nicotine gum. And that worked but I chewed the gum for three years. And I was still like my friend who still wanted to smoke when in "thinking hard" mode. The romance with cigarettes, for me, was not over.

I eventually started smoking again via hanging out with friends who smoked.

But this was all before I'd even heard of Allen Carr's method of stopping smoking. I was definitely doing it with a "willpower" method, one that requires a lot of willpower. I'd quit, but I still wanted it. I hadn't 'stopped'.

People who read this and Allen Carr's book are better able to cope with being with friends who smoke. Because they have dealt with the psychological addiction. They don't want to smoke anymore. I can be around friends who smoke now, and it isn't a big temptation for me to smoke, usually. There's a little stirring from time to time of a desire to smoke when I'm around them, but it isn't anything like an 'urge'. It's a kind of an irrational twinge that I observe in me. I observe it and appreciate my freedom. I enjoy my freedom from smoking. I am grateful and proud to be a non-smoker. I observe that I'm glad it's them smoking, not me. *Smoking is more enjoyable when someone else is doing it.*

You would also be well advised to say very little about your experience of stopping smoking, to your friends who smoke—unless they ask. If you want to help them stop smoking, you can do that mostly by example, not by talking. If you are able to hang out with them without wanting to smoke, they will notice that and eventually ask questions. Because of course smokers are afraid that if they try to stop they will still want to smoke and they will feel envious of smokers smoking. They will notice that you aren't envious of their smoking. If you are envious of their smoking, you're still hooked; you want one.

Stopping smoking is not something you can do for somebody else. Smokers must come to the decision on their own. You can't help them, except by example, before then. They will resent you, if you try, before they have made up their own mind.

47 - Addiction

Addiction is all about desire and illusion. Desire because you desire something, gotta have it, even in the face of terrible consequences. Illusion because it's like smoke, it's like dreams, hallucinations, the perfect escape, the intensest pleasure; and because, in addition to the illusions you know about, it comes with so many more that you just don't want to know about.

48 - Desire

When a smoker has a cigarette, they are happy because they are without desire for another cigarette.

> People confuse the source of their happiness. They become temporarily happy when they get a new car, or a new house, or a new marriage. And they think that they are suddenly happy because of this new thing in their life. In reality, they are happy because for a brief moment, they are without desire. But then soon another desire comes along. And the search continues.
>
> Brandon Stanton
> Humans of New York

49 - The Forbidden

Telling people about the dangers of smoking, particularly young people, does nothing to discourage them from smoking if the implication is that it's daring to smoke. *Education* by tobacco companies about the dangers of smoking is simply an *enticement* to smoke masquerading as *education*. Cigarette companies *target* youth as customers; they do not *educate* them.

Forbidden things can have a strong allure. Forbidden fruit was what Adam and Eve reputedly ate; it caused them to be thrown out of heaven but gave them the gift of knowledge. They fell from grace, lost their state of innocence. That is what teenagers want. They're tired of being kids and want to lose their state of innocence (childhood) and be adult. The idea that smoking the forbidden cigarettes will help them get there is mistaken, but it is similar to how Adam and Eve 'grew up'. Many teenagers think that if it's good enough for Adam and Eve, it's good enough for them.

It's also an act of defiance, of asserting their will against those who have forbidden them to smoke. The act of smoking is meant by young people to show they are not bound to obedience. It is meant by them to be an act signaling their independence of mind, their maturity into adulthood.

It's ironic that this attempt to assert independence results in new chains that take time to shake off. But smoking tobacco does have this *forbidden* aspect to it, to young people, that draws the defiance of some youngsters.

They don't understand that they are being drawn in to addiction by the mythos of cigarettes. The idea that smoking will help them become adults needs replacing. They need a better idea of what it means to become an adult. The rest of this chapter is addressed to kids.

The decisions of an adult don't always coincide with what they want. They look at the welfare of not just themselves but others. And adults don't do things just out of peer pressure or simply out of anger and defiance. Adults take a longer look before they act. Adults don't get suckered so easily into starting smoking. You don't see adults taking up smoking. Because it's a terrible decision, one of the worst you can make. Smokers themselves will tell you that.

The idea that smoking can help you is mistaken. It's forbidden to youngsters because it's poisonous and will eventually kill you. It doesn't help you with anything. It's a con.

There is no pill or product that can turn you into an adult. Only time will do that. Time and developing good judgment over time. Taking up smoking shows bad judgment, not good judgment. It's something tobacco companies want you to take up before you reach adulthood —because then you're far less likely to take it up. So taking up smoking is typically the decision of a child, not an adult. People will sell you a pill or a puff for all sorts of problems they don't help with. To take your money and hook you so they can keep taking your money.

The adult course of action on this matter is to avoid smoking. It only hurts you. It doesn't help you with anything. The adult thing to do is not to bow to peer pressure to start smoking, not to delude yourself that it helps you be cool or tough or bad ass or anything but a sucker sucking on poison. Whoever is advising you to take it up doesn't have your best interests at heart, on this matter. Smokers often like others to smoke too because it validates their addiction.

One of the important lessons in becoming an adult is to *avoid* smoking and other drugs. It may seem like taking it up will help make you older, more of an adult, because it's something only adults are allowed to do. But, in reality, deciding *not to take up smoking* is the adult thing to do. Not taking up smoking helps you become an adult more than starting smoking does.

It's very bad for you physically. But, also, it's bad for you mentally. Because it's a con job. You come to rely on it to give you help it doesn't give you. You're the one providing the help. Not the cigarettes. It's like thanking a swindler for the financial help he's supplying you with. When he's stealing your money, not helping you. You think the cigarettes help you deal with stress, but all they do is relieve the discomfort of withdrawal symptoms from nicotine. You think they help you concentrate, but they only relieve the distraction they themselves cause via withdrawal symptoms.

So it's interestingly different than the situation for Adam and Eve. They gained the gift of knowledge by eating the forbidden fruit. But youngsters learn more from *avoiding* smoking than they do from *taking it up*. Real education for youngsters about smoking is not to tell them not to smoke "because I told you so," but to let them in on the real nature of the addiction.

All their lives, they're going to have people trying to sell them things that are supposed to help them but don't. It starts in childhood; look at the awful food and snacks marketed to children. Only this is a little more serious because once people reach adulthood it's OK to sell them poison if they'll buy it. Not that all those sugary processed 'foods' for kids aren't poison too—many of them made by companies owned by tobacco companies[23].

---

23 See Michael Moss's book *Salt Sugar Fat—How the Food Giants Hooked Us*

50 - Restructure Your Breaks

There is a popular myth that smoking is for rebels. Rebellion is about attaining freedom. Smoking is about attaining servitude, being a slave to addiction. Rebellion is about fighting the status quo. Smoking is about paying lots of money to a wicked corporation that kills people for profit. Rebellion is resistance to consumerism. Smoking is about toxic, addicted consumption—the very *epitome* of negative consumerism.

Still, many smokers are rebels nonetheless. The usual form their rebellion takes is smoking as a break from all the demands on their time and attention that the world makes. Many people have to work hard at tasks that they would rather not have to spend so much time doing. They work hard, so they value their smoke-breaks. This is the only time they can say *no* to the work demands on them. Their smoking is their rebellion against all those demands on them.

This is a very serious issue for many smokers to deal with. If you're in this situation, you really need to know how to re-structure your breaks so that you don't have to smoke but you get what you need. If you don't deal with this issue effectively, you will probably go back to smoking. So let's look at this issue carefully and clearly. First, though, let me tell you about a friend of mine who was in this situation.

The first smoker I gave Allen Carr's book read it with great interest and stopped smoking during my visit east with her and her husband. Both of them are dear friends. She and I talked a lot that visit. She told me about how smoking was important to her as a break from taking care of her grand kids. She was saddled with taking care of a lot of demanding small children pretty much all day, most days. She is way too accommodating to her kids and their kids than to say no.

The only break she gets from it is when she goes outside to have a cigarette. They don't follow her when she smokes. She's outside on the back porch—rain or snow—so it isn't all that comfortable for her (or them) and of course she's smoking. Standing up. No chair. But she treasures those breaks.

And that's what drew her back to smoking after our visit. She lasted about a week before she started smoking again. It was those smoking breaks that got her going again. She didn't feel taking a break without smoking was an acceptable sort of break. Perhaps because then it would be clear she was taking the break to get some respite from the kids, rather than simply because she needed to service her addiction.

But, probably more importantly, she didn't know how to relax standing outside without smoking. How can you learn to relax without having a cigarette during your breaks? That's an important question.

First, we need to understand what is involved in being able to relax while having a cigarette.

There are two main things to consider. First, there's the matter of getting a nicotine fix, which temporarily alleviates withdrawal symptoms. That lets smokers temporarily feel like a normal person, who doesn't experience nicotine withdrawal symptoms. In your first week of stopping smoking, you'll still experience withdrawal symptoms, but if you have gotten rid of the desire to smoke, for the most part, you won't experience big urges, just the slight hunger pangs of the sensation of nicotine withdrawal. And after the first week, you won't experience nicotine withdrawal.

Getting rid of withdrawal symptoms by smoking provides the illusion that you're relaxing because it's a relief to get the nicotine monkey temporarily off your back. But your heart-rate increases. If you haven't had a cigarette for a day, you may need to sit down. You are not so much relaxed as slightly incapacitated, forced into less physical activity. You're ingesting a cocktail of cancerous poisons that hit you over the head. That is not relaxation. That saps your strength.

Relaxation, on the contrary, can be truly energizing and allow you to recoup your strength, rather than sapping it. The relaxation smokers experience in their smoke-breaks is not only from getting a nicotine fix; it's also from their conviction that they are getting some relaxation. Despite the fact that smoking a cigarette does more to make you feel worse than better, the mind is determined to wrest some relaxation from the smoke-break and does so quite successfully.

Imagine if your breaks were *genuinely* relaxing and vitalizing in addition to your mental relaxation. All along, you've been the one— not the cigarette—providing you with the relaxation. Giving the cigarette credit for your relaxation is like giving a freeloader vampire who sups on your neck credit for your relaxation.

You've been accepting an awful substitute for vitalizing relaxation—but you got one thing very right: you know how to relax mentally. The proof is you've been giving that to yourself all along. The cigarettes haven't been giving it to you. All they've been giving you is physical relief from withdrawal and the slight stupefaction of their minor intoxication.

How do you make your breaks relaxing and *better* than they were when you smoked?

Breathing exercises and muscle relaxation techniques can be an immense help and change for you. Learn about these and take what you learn to your breaks. Practice.

Also, if we're talking about breaks at your work-place, check out how the non-smokers there conduct their breaks. Also, there may be some infrastructure in place to help you, as a non-smoker, get what you need during your breaks.

Approach this matter of restructuring your breaks as a kind of a home improvement—with lots of creative energy, in any case. You're not just making a change. You're making a crucial change for the better. You're restructuring to create *better* breaks. You're learning how to *really* relax, not taking a drug for something that a drug can't give you. You are creating breaks where you get an infusion of *life force*, of *prana*, of revitalizing energy and relaxation.

The aspect of rebellion in the smoke-break is about taking control of your life. The saying *no* to all the demands on you is about exercising control over your life. Marlboro is all about a space that's free of all the demands and controls of contemporary civilization.

Of course, it's ironic that you use an addictive cigarette to attain that freedom and that rebellion from the status quo, that flight from control by all life's demands. It is a flight into the arms of a different and surely more sinister control: addiction to smoking and dependence on tobacco companies.

So you're restructuring your breaks not only to get better relaxation and re-energizing, but to attain freedom. Freedom from nicotine addiction. Freedom from fealty to the Mordor corporation that sells you cigarettes. Freedom from the painful irony of finding freedom in the servitude of addiction.

You need to approach this problem seriously and solve it. If you don't, you're probably going to go back to smoking. You need your best, most creative and enduring work on this one.

Think of your trigger situations—the situations surrounding your break that most give you the *time for a cigarette* signal and change those situations or create substitutes for smoking in them if you can't change the situation. You don't need a substitute for something you don't want, as I've said repeatedly earlier. But it doesn't hurt to remove or minimize or alter those trigger situations or your response to them.

Get some breathing exercises and possibly other exercises working for you in those break situations. Breathing exercises can help you with stress and relaxation much better than smoking can.

Also, you might have room in your breaks to introduce a bit of activity that you've previously said you always wanted to do but never had the time.

You need to solve this issue creatively. By thinking about what you really enjoy in life and how you can bring that closer to you in your breaks. Also, by creating a different situation than normally applies to your breaks.

If you hang out with smokers during your breaks, try to change that, at least for a few months. Over time, you are less and less interested in being around smoking. You become about as interested in being around smoking as you are in being around toxic waste. It is indeed toxic. And smoke is indeed waste.

51 - Early Tobacco Use

Tobacco came originally from the Andes around Peru in South America. There are some fascinating books on the history of tobacco such as Jordan Goodman's book *Tobacco in History — The Cultures of Dependence:*

> Amerindians (natives to the Americas) have been using tobacco for 3000-5000 years. When the Europeans arrived in the Americas in 1492, the natives were already smoking it, chewing it (snuff), drinking it, ingesting it as a jelly and taking enemas with it. The smoking of it was via pipes and also cigars.

Other scholars date smoking earlier to 9,000 years ago or, in other words, 7,000 BC:

> Because it is dependent on human propagation, *Nicotiana rustica* [one of two domesticated tobacco species] must have been taken north more than 7,000 miles, from the slopes of the Andes all the way to southern Canada, perhaps as the seeds were passed from one Indian to another, traveling at the rate of only a mile or less per year. Therefore, it is not unreasonable that it took 6,000 or 7,000 years for humans to spread the range of domesticated tobacco, beginning around 7000 B.C. If not earlier, until it reached the upper Mississippi Valley no later than A.D. 160[24].

Tobacco was used widely throughout the Americas from Alaska to South America. Even populations that did not cultivate any other plants, such as the Haida and Tlingit on Canada's west coast, grew it. It was often used very differently than it is now, but it was indeed used *very* widely throughout Amerindian nations and cultures. It had a wide range of functions and roles in Native cultures.

> What made tobacco unique among New World plants was that its effects were largely predictable, relatively

---

24 *Tobacco Use by Native North Americans*, Joseph C. Winter ed, U of Oklahoma Press, 2000, p.310

short-lived and not life-threatening (as datura could be) and thus had a vast functional repertoire. Its uses ranged from the purely symbolic to the medicinal; from its role as a hallucinogen in shamanistic practice and ritual to ceremonial and formal social functions; from profane to religious use; from its identification with myth and the supernatural to the formal ritualism of social experiences....

Tobacco's main function was to induce hallucinations in shamanistic rituals. It may seem surprising to find tobacco in this role, but it is important to recognize that there are big differences between the way tobacco was used then and now. First of all, it is certain that the species of tobacco used were *Nicotiana rustica* and *Nicotiana tabacum* or varieties of them. *Nicotiana tabacum* was generally used south of Mexico and *Nicotiana rustica* north of that country. Whatever the species, there is little doubt that the nicotine content was many times greater than that of present-day commercial species and varieties, and that it was capable, by itself, of inducing hallucinations. There is also some evidence that alkaloids other than nicotine are present in non-commercial varieties. These may be hallucinogenic in their own right, and possibly even more so in combination with high concentrations of nicotine. Finally, there is also some evidence that tobacco was often mixed with other more potent substances. Growing evidence leaves little doubt that at the time of contact, tobacco was valued primarily for its psychoactive powers, especially since they were mild when compared to other substances.[25]

As we know, tobacco, as it's currently used, is *not* hallucinogenic. So it's surprising to learn that it was precisely that to the Amerindians. It was a hallucinogen in shamanistic rituals. That means the drug was

---

25 *Tobacco in History*, Part I: "Food of the Spirits — Shamanism, healing and tobacco in Amerindian cultures", p.24-25, Jordan Goodman, 1993, Routledge

used by the shaman to travel in the spirit world. Shamanic rituals often involved healing. Amerindians believed that the causes of many illnesses were supernatural. The uses of tobacco by the shamans in healing were multiple. They used it as a hallucinogen to travel in the spirit world; they would use it in the diagnosis process, sometimes blowing mouthfuls of smoke on the body of the victim to locate the afflicted region, and the prescription was often some form of tobacco as well. Tobacco was used as a medication for everything under the sun.

Although modern tobacco is not typically hallucinogenic and it's not typically used in the contemporary world in shamanistic healing rituals, this history is not without relevance to the current situation although there are big differences.

We see that the addiction is 99% psychological and that dismantling that psychological dependence involves looking closely at a set of illusions that are dear to smokers. These are not *hallucinations* that the smoker experiences, but we are still dealing with a field of dreams, as it were. The drug still operates in a way that provides the user with convincing illusions, primarily via the withdrawal symptoms its use initiates. The illusions, in the modern world, are the typical ones we're familiar with: smoking is enjoyable, helps reduce stress, is good for concentration, relaxation, tastes good, and so on.

Also, the Amerindians used tobacco as medication. Doctors such as Vancouver's Dr. Gabor Maté believe that all addictions, fundamentally, are attempts to self-medicate traumatic experiences from the past, typically from early childhood. The idea is that the compulsive behavior is an attempt to assuage the strong fears and insecurities (amplifiers of the mild physical dependence) that traumatic emotional pain has caused. The carefully cultivated public image of tobacco is associated with the calming of fears, calming of nerves, with a little escape from whatever is going on.

In actuality, it provides only relief from the withdrawal symptoms that it itself causes, rather than providing any genuine calming influence. In fact, after you have a cigarette, the nicotine soon starts to cause agitation, not calmness. It provides more agitation than calming because it perpetuates a cycle of agitation followed by calming of that very agitation. Still, the illusion that it's a calming drug is felt to be convincing because the temporary relief smoking provides from withdrawal symptoms is real. This is the sort of illusion that the drug does well. The illusion that tobacco has psychological medicinal properties such as inducing calmness is one that is notoriously convincing until you look closely at it, at which point the illusion dissolves like smoke.

52 - The Progress of Tobacco in History

Consider the awesome history of tobacco. Originating in the New World, tobacco was the most widely used drug among Amerindians from Alaska to Argentina, from the land of the Haida on the west coast to eastern Canada. It was venerated by the Amerindians for its purported wide medicinal capabilities and, among other things, it was used by shamans to enter and travel in the spirit world via its hallucinogenic(!) properties.

When the Europeans arrived in the Americas, they quickly began exporting tobacco to all corners of the globe and praised tobacco as a medicinal panacea capable of curing a multitude of afflictions including cancers.

How does it come to be that a herb of such apparently surpassing medicinal excellence is the greatest single cause of preventable deaths in the world, annually killing 5 million people (the population of Finland) from a panoply of fatal diseases brought about through persistent use of this highly addictive ex-hallucinogen? How did such a killer—'serial killer' doesn't really begin to cover it—serial killers are pikers compared with the numbers of people tobacco kills—get confused with a panacea?

It isn't the only time that a drug that we now think of as dangerous was hailed originally for its medicinal value. Cocaine and heroin were touted in the 19th century as *wonder drugs*. Sigmund Freud was very enthusiastic about cocaine. He prescribed it extensively and was himself addicted.

The early history of heroin goes something like this:

> Diacetyl morphine was first discovered in 1874 in St Mary's Hospital, London, and traded after 1899 by Bayer under the trade name 'Heroin'. This was a more powerful painkiller than morphine, yet in the early twentieth century it was still considered a gentle medicine to be used mainly against respiratory symptoms. In Europe, it was initially heralded as a chemically pure, non-addictive anesthetic, and was also widely used as an effective remedy for morphine addiction. In the 1900's heroin was widely applied

hypodermically as a non-addictive substitute for morphine by doctors in Europe and the United States. Pharmaceutical companies marketed it as a cure for numerous diseases, including infantile respiratory ailments, coughs and bronchitis.[26]

The wonder drug of its generation heralded for its medicinal excellence—imagine giving infants "non-addictive" heroin—sometimes emerges in the next generation as a dangerous and outlawed substance. Such was the case with heroin and cocaine. The drawbacks of drugs are usually not as quickly apparent as the benefits, and the benefits often recede with continued usage.

But tobacco has not undergone the fate of heroin or cocaine. While it's regulated, to some extent, in most countries, it is available to adults legally. There isn't a country in the world, presently, that has made it illegal to adults.

Tobacco is a much more polite killer than cocaine or heroin. It does not create a confused or stoned user. Even when it does, that doesn't last long. The withdrawal symptoms are unlike the relatively extreme physical unpleasantness associated with alcohol, heroin, and cocaine withdrawal. Smoking can even be made to look good, as we see in old movies. The health effects usually develop slowly, over the course of decades, almost imperceptibly at first. Tobacco is a relatively refined and sophisticated—although quite efficient—killer. One in two smokers will die prematurely of smoking-related illnesses.

These factors and many others have created a history in which, as Jordan Goodman puts it, "...tobacco has become a universal addiction for consumers, for growers and for governments":

> The main concern of this book is to explain how humankind became involved with the tobacco plant, and how the relationships between it and ourselves have changed over time....the history of tobacco is full of conflict, compromise, coercion and co-operation. It is through this historical process that tobacco has become a universal addiction for consumers, for growers and for governments.

> Indeed, this is the overall theme of the book.

---

26 p. 155 from Narcotic Culture—A history of drugs in China

Dependence unifies the history of tobacco whether seen from the vantage point of the consumer, of the producer or of the institutions concerned with its promulgation....Shamans depended on tobacco's unique pharmacological properties as they themselves became dependent upon it through its addictive powers. Under European control early colonial settlement became dependent upon tobacco and early settlers were addicted both as consumers and as producers to the culture of the plant. Governments, too, have become dependent on the tax revenue they derive by controlling its distribution....This multi-faceted structure of dependence is what makes the history of tobacco fascinating while explaining why it has become so deeply entrenched throughout the world.[27]

Governments the world over are as hooked as smokers—not on *nicotine*, but on the *revenue* generated by tobacco. Napoleon (1808-73) quipped: "This vice brings in one hundred million francs in taxes every year. I will certainly forbid it at once—as soon as you can name a virtue that brings in as much revenue."

---

27 Goodman, p.13-14

53 - Addictionism

It isn't just individuals who get addicted to nicotine. As Jordan Goodman points out in *Tobacco in History – The Cultures of Dependence*, dependence on tobacco by growers and at the state level—states have been addicted to revenue from tobacco for hundreds of years--"unifies the history of tobacco" in "cultures of dependence".

Some would argue that health care systems exhibit dependence also. There is a huge industry devoted to treating the diseases caused by smoking. The high cost of this industry to the state—this cost is higher than the revenue from tobacco—is one of the prime motivators for the state to deal with its addiction to tobacco.

Also, nicotine substitutes such as gums and patches wean smokers, at least temporarily, away from smoking but leave them with a nicotine addiction and untreated psychological dependence. They're still very reliable customers, but the product has changed to a 'healthier' one within the health care system.

Addictive products are impervious to economic downturns and many of the vicissitudes of history. While consumers, in hard times, may spend less on some products because money is tight, addicts cough up the cash for their addictions come what may. Addictive products make for profitable, dependable businesses.

That is a strong factor in any culture, be it capitalist or communist. Addictionism transcends capitalism and communism. Tobacco is at least as big a problem in China and all the former Soviet states as it is in the west; there are in excess of 300,000,000 smokers in China, possibly more than the entire population of the USA. And if you look at the statistics concerning tobacco use per capita[28], communist or formerly communist countries such as Serbia, Bulgaria, Russia, Moldova, Ukraine, Slovenia, Bosnia and Herzegovina, Belarus, the Czech Republic, Kazakhstan and Azerbaijan were all in the top 16 countries in the world in 2015.

I remember looking at Russian posters from the time of the

---

28 See
en.wikipedia.org/wiki/List_of_countries_by_cigarette_consumption_per_capita for a list of countries ranked by cigarette consumption per capita.

communist revolution in 1917. There were a few with cigarette ads on them.

Addictionism is about providing people in distress with medicine. But it doesn't help them with their distress; it addicts them into being the most reliable customers on the planet. It's a kind of economic and ideological taxation and servitude that cuts across communist and capitalist states.

Even the contemporary market for videogames is sprinkled with the rhetoric of addiction. Good games, it's said, have that 'addictive' quality. I used to think it would be wonderful to write the world's first addictive poem—as a computer game/poem. But now I feel that trying to make anything be addictive is not about making good art. Good art helps us free ourselves from chains. Hooking people addictively is about exploiting their insecurities. You're just making another consumer product in the ideology of addictionism.

In ridding yourself of your addiction to smoking, you are also ridding yourself of being a supporter of global addictionism which is unthinkingly supported by tobacco addicts around the world and embraced by the global businesses that minister both to the desire for nicotine and the dire health effects it has on millions around the world. Addictionism is desire and illusion that drives economies in mindless consumerism toward ill health decades down the line in a generational cycle.

The cure for individuals and society involves education. Education about the nature of psychological addiction and how to deal with it effectively. And education about how addiction functions as something that happens not only to individuals but at a societal level. And, of course, education about the costs to society and individuals of tobacco addiction; that is a dialog that has successfully been underway in the west for several decades.

54 - Ancient and Modern

A *tabaquero*, a tobacco-using shaman in Ecuador, was quoted as saying "One of the secrets of tobacco is that the less you use, the more powerful it is."

Smokers know that if they go without a cigarette for a day or more then, when they have one, they get dizzy and walloped by their cigarette. The physical effect is stronger that way. That's one of the meanings of what the tabaquero said. But, additionally, the withdrawal symptoms have been annoying for some time, for smokers who forgo a cigarette for some time, and so when they finally do have a cigarette, the psychological relief is strong. They are dizzy, walloped, and relieved of their withdrawal symptoms that have built up like Chinese water torture. They don't normally hallucinate, but they are stoned for a minute—but only a minute, and then return quickly to normal form. That is another meaning of what the shaman said.

If you haven't had a cigarette for quite a while, the smoke hits your system like a frying pan gonged off the top of your skull. You would like to sit down. You're shaky on your feet. Your heart is pounding. You are stupefied. If you were sad, you are now not thinking about it. If you were worried, it has slipped your mind. If you were stressed, well, now your heart is pounding, but the relief from no more withdrawal symptoms is *such* a relief.

You know it's poison, at that point. The body's reaction tells you unequivocally that it's distressed. But the cessation of withdrawal symptoms is such a relief that, together with the walloping and dizziness, it almost seems like bliss.

But the shaman may have had additional power in mind. If you want but cannot or do not have something for a long time, and then you have it, you 'receive it like a sacrament', to borrow a phrase. The genuinely religious experiences of indigenous peoples around tobacco would be heightened when tobacco use was something for special occasions, rather than a pack-a-day thing.

But it also puts strain on nicotine addicts to be without their drug that long. If someone is addicted to nicotine, then just because they only have one cigarette per day does not mean they are not Jonesing for a cigarette worse than those who smoke 20 or more per day. Regular smokers who only smoke a few per day are often struggling quite hard to maintain that low level of consumption. It's a difficult struggle. When they have a cigarette, they almost feel they're at heaven's gate, they're so relieved. Amen? Amen. But of course that sort of relief requires a lot of preliminary suffering. Which is often a serious problem for those who smoke regularly but not very much.

Further, they are as hooked as anyone else. Perhaps even more so in that, as the shaman, says, "One of the secrets of tobacco is that the less you use, the more powerful it is." The less you use it and yet remain a regular, addicted user, the more lovely it seems when you have one, the more convinced you are of its valuable aid, and so on.

Nicotine addiction involves a kind of hunger. Not hunger for food but for nicotine. Ah but smokers will say "I don't think of it as a hunger for nicotine but for cigarettes." It can come in many shapes and sizes. As long as it's full of nicotine.

We hunger for food, we hunger for sex, we hunger for intimacy, for love, for acceptance, and for success. Smoking and the hunger it brings naturally gets involved with our psychic hungers. Some feel that their cigarettes are their dependable little friend who's always there for them. Smoking for some people gives them sexual pleasure; they have a kind of sexual relationship with smoking. Others feel it calms them down better than a good counselor. There's a strong relationship smokers have with smoking, with their cigarettes/tobacco/nicotine. There's a romance.

The indigenous peoples of the Americas often thought of tobacco as the food of the Spirits and the hunger we feel for nicotine as a Spirit's hunger for tobacco. The addiction, in that case, is not an addiction, but *a hunger by Spirits* for their real food: tobacco. We are not addicted to (real) food—though we may be addicted to overeating. If the food of the spirits is tobacco and we feel their hunger, we are not addicted but simply feeling their hunger for their proper food. How's that for a completely different point of view on nicotine addiction?

If the hunger of addiction is experienced as the hunger of the Spirits, then that hunger is a religious experience; in such cultures, tobacco is not an addiction but a religious experience; the pangs of addiction are experienced as the very hunger of the spirits.

Tobacco was deeply important to the religion of many tribes. You would expect big differences concerning tobacco between such cultures and cultures where tobacco is simply a recreational drug. Even if it's used recreationally in a culture in which tobacco is sacred, it might and probably would still have some sort of religious residue, some residue as a religious experience, in this case of the hunger of the Spirits. They themselves speak of experiencing that hunger. To non-Natives, it's a nicotine addiction, withdrawal symptoms of a nicotine addiction. To Natives, it's a religious experience of the hunger of the Spirits. BIG difference.

People in such native cultures conceive of the act of smoking as feeding the hungry spirit its proper food.

Additionally, among many native peoples, to offer the spirits tobacco or to smoke it is to give the spirits a gift that they cannot refuse. And it's a gift that the spirits must give you something in return for. They want tobacco more than anything, so they will give you what you want for it.

This is more familiar. In non-Native cultures, smoking is used to 'make everything better'—or at least to make you feel better, to relieve tension, stress, worry, fear, anxiety.

Even though smoking is rarely hallucinogenic, it's nonetheless wrapped up in desire and illusion. In native cultures in which tobacco is important, smoking is often conceived as an act that will actually make things better in that the spirits will fulfill one's request. That isn't so terribly different from the expectations smokers in non-Native cultures have of smoking. They too smoke to obtain from smoking benefits that smoking does not really provide. But the relief one experiences from withdrawal symptoms (that smoking causes) when one smokes is enough to convince people that smoking helps them feel better, whatever was ailing them, often.

55 - The Attraction of Smoking in a Stressful Situation

> A few miles away they're incinerating
> the haystacks and the houses,
> while squatting here on the fringe of this
> pleasant meadow,
> the shell-shocked peasants quietly smoke their
> pipes....

That's a poem called "Postcard 2" by the Hungarian poet Miklós Radnóti written in 1944 during World War II. The "peasants" whose houses and haystacks are being incinerated can do nothing about it. Smoking is the only satisfaction they will get that day, if any, if they were not shot by the retreating Hungarian army.

When we're sad, worried or ill and can do basically nothing to cure the situation, a drug that will at least distract us from our problems and offer some temporary relief can be attractive.

The drug offers relief from withdrawal symptoms in the guise of pleasure, but for those in a situation where satisfactions of any kind are few and far between, and sadness, worry, and misery are the order of the day, trading pleasure for relief may seem like a no-brainer as long as it does indeed bring some relief. If the future looks bleak anyway, how much worse can a nicotine addiction be? If it at least provides some short-term satisfaction, then it may seem entirely worth the bargain—whatever it may be.

You have been down related roads before. But now it's different. You understand that once you get over the physical addiction, smoking doesn't even provide relief from withdrawal symptoms. When you're over the physical addiction, a desire for a cigarette is pure psychological addiction. You know smoking doesn't give you any of the important things you thought it gave you. You don't really even want one. There's just nothing in it for you. The cigarette company is the only one profiting from it.

So what is it that you want? A cigarette or something else? It's something else, isn't it. You want something to feel better. But all smoking has for you are empty illusions of medicinal value. And, of course, lots of negative things.

This can be of considerable help to you in rough situations. Because it's an affirmation of the truth about smoking, and a rejection of smoking based on getting to the heart of the psychological addiction. When you're in a rough situation, you can be proud that you have not only made your way without smoking, but you've come to a better understanding of yourself and what you want. You can't fool yourself quite so easily anymore; you don't want to fool yourself about smoking. Or anything else.

When the heat is on and you find you don't even want a cigarette, be proud and get on with your life.

56 - Freedom

How does it feel to be a non-smoker after you've been a smoker? You feel the joy of one who is no longer inadvertently but inexorably killing yourself. You're free from an oppression that has killed millions of people. If you live in places where smoking is largely banned, you feel relief from having to isolate yourself from others. And you're free from supporting monstrous corporations to poison you and others. You are free from the triumph of matter over mind.

It's a relief and cause for joy, hope, and strong feelings of well-being.

It's OK to feel those things. In fact it's important to be able to feel that joy, relief, and happiness every time you feel the dying remnant of your desire for a cigarette. Rejoice in your new-found freedom, feel the joy, relief and happiness of it in your heart. You have earned it by freeing yourself from smoking.

Every time you think you want a cigarette, get in touch with your own joy, rightful pride at having cured yourself of this addiction, and feel the well-being so dearly earned and know that the inclination to smoke is dying in you. What you will have instead is the song in your heart you feel even now as you liberate yourself from addiction. That's the feeling of freedom from addiction. Treasure it. Your joy and freedom. Gotta love it. It's a permanent relief, not something temporarily acquired by smoking poison.

It's the feeling of being freed from a terrible addiction. The relief smoking gave you was temporary: relief from withdrawal symptoms caused also by smoking. The relief from withdrawal symptoms you have now achieved can be permanent. It couldn't feel better. It's the feeling of *real* relaxation, of *real* concentration, of *real* contentment and joy, of *real* freedom that you have earned. Earned by your understanding of what you thought smoking was giving you and your understanding that it does not give you those things. Earned by ending the romance with smoking.

To free yourself from the addiction to smoking is not simply a way to greater physical health, although it certainly is that, and in a very big way. Additionally, in coming to understand the nature of the addiction, in disabusing yourself of the illusions that the addiction relies on, you have freed your mind in a significant way. This does not solve all your problems and guarantee you live happily ever after, but it's a big and important change in your life—and a very positive one. You have a knowledgeable consciousness of the power of illusion in cigarette addiction. These probably won't be the only illusions you will now begin to question and debunk, knowing now, as you do, something of how that game works.

You have freed your own mind of some serious illusions. You have dared to open your mind. You don't have to lie to yourself anymore about smoking. You don't have to pretend it tastes good. You don't have to pretend you enjoy them. You don't have to give cigarettes credit for your concentration powers. You don't have to lie to yourself about anything to do with smoking. That makes you less tolerant of lying to yourself more generally. You are a little less vulnerable to falsehoods, propaganda, lies, and just plain bullshit. From others. And from yourself to yourself.

When you stop smoking, there's a period of about a week before the physical addiction is finished. During this time, if you have debunked your illusions about smoking, you won't feel any cravings to smoke. However, you need to know how to deal with the dying twinges of what Allen Carr calls "the little monster". To Carr, "the little monster" is the physical addiction. The "big monster" is the psychological addiction.

You don't feel cravings anymore for cigarettes, but you do feel the pathetic death twinges of the little monster. As you know all too well, the addiction to nicotine has established a schedule of feeding the little monster nicotine, whereupon it goes to sleep but then wakes up and irritates you until you feed it again.

How do you deal with those little proddings of your dying physical addiction? You rejoice in your new found freedom. You experience real enjoyment. If you're not feeling urges to smoke but only the pathetic mild hunger pangs of the little monster, you'll be plenty happy and will enjoy the situation immensely. You have rid yourself of a blood sucking vampire on your neck. You are no longer in servitude to an addiction that was hurting you and hurting those around you. You are free of it. Feel it. Enjoy it.

Breathe deeply. Soon you will not be hacking and coughing. Your lungs will begin to clear up almost immediately and will continue to get better for years.

Enjoy your relief from the suffering that is smoking. But you have more than relief from suffering to enjoy and look forward to. You have the many health benefits you can look forward to enjoying. But, moreover, you also have won your freedom from captivity by a monster. You have freed your mind. You now know what it means to free your mind, if you didn't before. It turns out that freeing your mind is the crucial achievement in stopping smoking. Seeing through illusions is the main task. Coming to understand the truth is the main thing. The truth does indeed set you free, in this case.

You have penetrated to the other side of the darkness. You have seen the light. I'm not talking about religious ecstasy. I'm talking about the freedom of mind that takes you out of the hands of a painful addiction that was slowly killing you.

Being free from it is cause for joy. Feel that joy. Every time the little monster makes an appearance, you need to practice feeling that joy. You'll get good at it very soon. And you can carry on with it after the physical addiction is over. That's important.

A friend of mine, one time when I was down in the dumps, said to me "Let's play a little game, you and me. Let's have a little race. But this is no typical race. The first one to feel happy wins. Ready? One two three GO!" We both laughed. "I'd say it was a tie," he said.

When that little monster growls its weaselly little growl, you just rejoice in your hard won, long sought freedom and all the good things that go with it. It's good practice to enjoy life more. And you surely can enjoy life more now that you have retired those illusions, traded them for the truth, freed your mind from poisonous lies, and freed your body from poisonous toxins.

Feel that joy every day. Don't let a day go by from now until the day you die without feeling the joy of this freedom you have won. It will defeat the little monster and bigger ones too.

57 - First Man and Sky Father

"Tobacco is woven throughout the mythology and the ceremonials" of Navajo culture, says Joseph C Winter (*Tobacco Use by Native North Americans*, U of Oklahoma Press, 2000, p.269). "Its critical importance is reflected by the fact that creation itself was brought about when Sky Father and Earth Mother smoked this sacred plant. Sky Father needed the smoke to think about the awesome task that lay ahead." Winter then quotes from a Navajo creation story:

> First Man had already guessed this. "All right, I see, so it is indeed," First Man said, "there should be tobacco for you!" That is called the wide leaf, the slender leaf, the dark-tipped and the white-tipped. "This will be your tobacco," he told Sky Father. "By this token it will become mutually known to us," he told him. "you see, in...occasion for sorrow (worry) at any time in your mind, you can smoke it!"

First Man tells Sky Father he can smoke tobacco any time Sky Father feels sorrow or worry. That's a common use of tobacco now. Tobacco has been used for a very long time to feel better when sadness or sorrow strike us. The way it works is this. Nicotine makes you suffer most of the time from withdrawal symptoms. Suffering from withdrawal symptoms becomes standard consciousness, normal, the usual state of mind. The mild hunger of withdrawal blends with the other perpetual hungers and dissatisfactions of modern life. But there is a cure for this particular hunger: smoke tobacco. Hunger solved.

You may not feel relief from your sadness, sorrow, anxiety, stress, or fear, but at least you feel relief from nicotine withdrawal.

It's a lousy deal. But even Sky Father falls for it from time to time. Like when he has an awesome task in front of him that he isn't sure he can handle. First Man to the rescue. First Man has something good for Sky Father. Something that will make Sky Father need First Man forever after. Something addictive. Something that will poison Sky Father and make him perpetually hungry for relief from the poison. The antidote happens to be more poison. That'll cheer him up.

Wow. That First Man was slick. And he wasn't the last, that's for sure. Sky Father better keep an eye on that one; he's slippery.

58 - Dependence

That tobacco was so widespread among the indigenous peoples of both North and South America at the time of European contact in 1492 is remarkable. It tells us some interesting things.

First, assuming people originally entered the Americas across the Bering land bridge, when Russia and Alaska were joined by land that has since been covered by ocean, they had to make their way from Alaska south to the Andes in Peru, where tobacco originates. That's a distance of about 7,000 miles. Researchers commonly use 1 mile per year as the average speed at which we can reasonably assume migration took place. So it takes 7,000 years just to migrate far enough south to where tobacco originates.

Then tobacco has to be adopted, smoked, and spread throughout the Americas, again at about 1 mile per year. It's thought that people have been smoking tobacco anywhere from 5,000 to 9,000 years. The distance that it spread was, again, roughly 7,000 miles, from the northern Andes of Peru south throughout South America, but, more distantly, north to the eastern seaboard of the USA and Canada as well as to the west coast of Canada among the Haida and Tlingit. And more or less all points between.

Further, we know that tobacco spread by human contact, not via the wind and other natural processes, because the varieties that came to grow in North America require some human cultivation.

For tobacco to have spread as widely as it did, it seems that people would have had to have inhabited the Americas for at least 14,000 years. And, indeed, give or take a couple of thousand years, that is about how long many people think humans have been in the Americas, though some (hotly contested) evidence is starting to emerge that we may have been there for as long as 50,000 years.[29] And for tobacco to have spread about 7,000 miles, it would have had to have been cultivated for at least 7,000 years.

In any case, it's fascinating to think about how tobacco spread so successfully, so broadly in the Americas. Even among peoples who cultivated no other plants. How was this possible?

---

29 See the research of Dr. Albert Goodyear, for instance, at sciencedaily.com/releases/2004/11/041118104010.htm

Well, first, of course, it's physically addictive. And we know that the nicotine content was much higher. Which means it was even more physically addictive than today's commercial strains.

But we also know that the addiction to smoking is largely psychological. We're familiar with the mythos of smoking—the stories and assumptions—in *contemporary* culture; we know the reasons why young people turn to it, sometimes, in the mistaken hope that it will help them. And we know the stories adults tell themselves about what smoking does for them. But what about the mythos of tobacco in ancient Amerindian cultures?

Mythos was surely crucial also in the spread of tobacco. It spread not only as something people smoked, but as something offered to the spirits so that one's prayers would be heard and granted. It spread as the food of the spirits, something they craved above all else, something they would be very grateful for when offered to them by humans. It also spread as something that was supposed to have great healing powers for mortals. And it spread as something that was supposed to sooth worries and sadness. Additionally, the higher nicotine concentration is sometimes associated with hallucinations, catatonia (and sometimes death from overdoses), and shamans used tobacco to enter and travel through the spirit world.

Such was the original mythos of tobacco. Most of it sounds pretty good. It would be worth the nauseating initiation all smokers are familiar with. It would be something that not only children would take up as a matter of youthful folly, which is what happens now, but something adults would be willing to initiate into for its supposed important benefits. Smoking would even be a sign of piety in some cultures.

The mythos sounds too good to be true, and of course it is, but recall that European culture also embraced smoking as a panacea, a cure-all, an incredibly curative herb, for several hundred years. The indigenous peoples got tobacco with all the power of religion. The Europeans got it with medicine.

We see that the history of tobacco relies on our desire to believe tobacco and smoking can provide us with great and important things. That is true across the board, across time and cultures.

Tobacco has enjoyed phenomenal marketing from day one, then. The mythos of the indigenous peoples concerning tobacco is extremely attractive. Tobacco helps you get your wishes fulfilled when you offer it to the spirits. And, when smoked, it transports you to the spirit-realm. It was also supposed to be very powerful medicinally.

At least in the case of indigenous cultures, we can imagine the mythos as not being an evil concoction of jackals who know the harm they do but do it anyway as forcefully as possible. Instead, tobacco in the Americas spread with the force of religion, prayer, and humanity's fervent desire for relief from our afflictions.

Still, the spread of tobacco in the pre-contact Americas was not simply a matter of an addictive substance spread with religious fervor. Surely another reason for its successful spread was its value as an article of trade.

If you have tobacco and great stories about what it can do for someone, you've got something that might put food on the table. You've got an advantage in the trade if the customer is an addict and wants it badly.

Tobacco spread not only as an important gift of religious significance, but as something that could be successfully traded, something that could fetch a good price, especially after the customer was indoctrinated into tobacco's use and benefits, i.e, after they were hooked. It may sometimes have spread as something that gave one group power over another group. Until they too could grow their own. And then trade it with a group who couldn't.

There is a common belief that the religious use of tobacco by indigenous peoples spared them from addiction. But religion provides no special dispensation from addiction.

> Time and again, early [European] observers expressed their astonishment at the tobacco addiction of many of the Indians they met. Various peoples belonging to both the Iroquoian and Algonkian language families were seen with pipes in their mouths at all hours of the day and night, and tobacco figured prominently in the dreams they recalled....Occasionally, the natives themselves admitted that there was nothing in the world they loved more than tobacco....Paul Le Jeune reported that the fondness the Montagnais had for

tobacco was "beyond belief." They went to sleep with their pipes in their mouths, got up at night to smoke, [and] interrupted their journeys to do the same....[30]

Tobacco wasn't just used for religious events. It was also used more broadly, in a secular way. If it was used religiously to win favors from the spirits, who themselves craved it beyond all else, it was also used to trade with neighboring tribes to win favors from them. Tobacco has been important in both spirituality and politics for a long time.

Jordan Goodman's book is titled *Tobacco in History—the Cultures of Dependence*. That phrase "the cultures of dependence" is crucial. Think of the spread of tobacco throughout the Americas as a tree structure with links of dependence. This tribe depended on that tribe for their tobacco. And then grew their own, eventually. And then passed it on to another tribe who, in turn, depended on them. Tobacco spread successfully because those links of dependence are not just strong by dint of the addictive power of tobacco—physically and psychologically—but also because the trading, the depending on one another, was important to keep them being friends and in touch with one another. To this day, trading partners are less likely to go to war with one another. Dependence made for enduring relationships and shared cultural and religious values between tribes.

Those sorts of dependencies in the fabric of tobacco dissemination have largely disappeared. What is left are big companies distributing a product to people they don't know and would rather not know, a product that has been emptied of its religious significance and is mostly an ineffective medicine for poor people to cope with their lot. It is less a medicine, now, than a vampirical and poisonous alternative to the panoply of modern anti-depressants, weight-loss pills, and so on.

Still, though, there's that magical belief people invest in it, belief that it is helping them cope. How much better for them to see that they themselves are the source of the strength that has allowed them to cope, and smoking is just dragging them down.

---

30 From *Tobacco Use by Native North Americans: Sacred Smoke and Silent Killer*, chapter 3 by Alexander von Gernet: "North American Indigenous Nicotiana Use and Tobacco Shamanism," p.74, p.78.

59 - Your Last Cigarette

If this book has worked for you, either you smoked your last cigarette some time ago, several pages ago, or it's time to do that now. If you still want to smoke, it hasn't worked yet. Because the idea is to get rid of your desire to smoke.

If you're thinking "Oh God I have to quit now", you're not done: you're hooked when you want one. The idea is to get rid of your desire to smoke.

If you agree that you don't enjoy smoking, the 'enjoyment' of smoking went out the window for you a while ago. You can't enjoy your last cigarette because you know you don't and never really did enjoy smoking.

By the time it's time to smoke your last cigarette, you're pretty much done, if we have connected as I hope we have and you're at the final stage of stopping smoking.

Part of what's involved in stopping smoking is developing a sense of observing how you really feel when you smoke a cigarette.

Is the romance of smoking over for you? There's an excitement of anticipation in the romance, a build-up to smoking so that the smoking comes as a great relief, almost like a little orgasm of relief. That's part of the amplifier. That excitement of anticipation amplifies the irritation of the withdrawal symptoms into an urge to smoke.

But when you've ended the romance, the thrill is gone. The thrill, the build up of desire and anticipation—you can recognize that's something you maintain like a romance. You can observe yourself and how you maintain it. And when you do, you can see also how you can put it aside. Because it's very much an abusive romance, and you're the one getting the abuse. You supply the thrill yourself; it isn't inherent in the drug or the activity.

Smoking has been as addictive as it has been for 9,000 years not because smoking is that fulfilling and pleasurable, but because it provides a plausible illusion of pleasure and fulfillment, and our deep need for pleasure and fulfillment does the rest, fills in the blank, even makes a romance with an inanimate drug, out of our deep needs.

If I ever get executed, and they ask me if I want a final cigarette—if they still do that, or ever did that—I doubt I'd want one. It would give me more pleasure to realize I didn't want one than to con myself with a lie that I did. Knowing that you don't want it, even or especially in times of stress, is a source of strength. In fact it's a greater source of strength than smoking is. And it isn't a matter of denying yourself something you want. You don't desire it or want it. The romance is over. The spell is over.

I used to drink alcohol to be able to deal with public occasions, sometimes. I thought it made me more fun and the events more fun. I used it to cope with some stressful situations. Of course, it wasn't a very good way of coping with them at all. Now I don't feel the need or desire to do that. I don't feel any need to cloak myself. I may not be particularly fun or interesting. But I'll be there just as me, and am interested to encounter other people just that way too. I don't feel the need to escape from those encounters into a more 'viable me'. In any case, alcohol doesn't provide a better me. It provides a worse.

Similarly, I don't feel that smoking helps me cope better with *anything* or that it provides a better me in *any* sense, really. I still have problems coping with things, sometimes. I still avoid and procrastinate. But at least I don't reach for a cigarette in the mistaken belief that it's going to do anything good for me.

Recreational drugs are overrated. Drugs that seem to start out as enhancers of parts of ourselves inevitably end up diminishing those and other parts of ourselves. They cater to our insecurities that we ourselves *aren't enough*. We aren't enough to be able to deal effectively with what we have to do. Or we aren't enough to be able to enjoy ourselves, or have other people enjoy us.

It's funny, but in fact we get better when we make the simple determination to just be ourselves and proceed without smoking or alcohol, and let the chips fall as they may—just on us being ourselves, warts and all. There's great strength in it. *You are enough just as you are.* And you can be proud that you know it. Don't listen to anyone who tells you otherwise.

If you still smoke, smoke that last cigarette, if you like. It isn't the moment before you're blindfolded and executed. *It's the moment before you walk free from a jail cell you've been locked in too long. You've got the key.*

60 - The 'Medicinal Value of Smoking'

Tobacco products used to be widely prescribed for a dizzying number of ailments. In the west they are no longer prescribed by doctors for *any* ailments. The medicinal value of smoking is near 0. It's like the medicinal value of nuclear bombs. Great for population control but there are serious side effects.

It does have some medicinal value, though. It's a great pesticide, makes bugs want to get away from you or even kills them because nicotine is seriously poisonous not only to humans but insects also. Nicotine and especially neonicotinoids, chemicals derived from nicotine, are widely used as pesticides. Imidacloprid, a neonicotinoid, is the most widely used insecticide in the world. Neonicotinoids are also thought to be strongly related to the problem with the drop in number of bees around the world.

Smoking used to be prescribed as a means of weight-control because, for some people, it suppresses hunger. Many others find that they eat more when they smoke. Killing yourself is a very effective means of weight-control, if somewhat extreme. So too is smoking as a means of weight-control. There are better means out there, even if it works for you as a weight-control factor.

In any case, the idea that you will gain weight when you stop smoking applies only if you substitute eating for smoking. But our approach does not require substitutes: *you don't need a substitute for something you don't want.*

The idea that smoking has medicinal value is a *very old* misconception. Some would be less kind and say it's an outright lie or even a mountainous pile of bs. It's important to get a sense of how large that mountain is and why it's so huge.

First, how old is this mountain? It's thought that people have been smoking in the Americas for about 5,000-9,000 years. When Europeans first sailed to the Americas, tobacco, already for thousands of years, had been widely used by the indigenous peoples as one of their most sacred spiritual and medicinal plants. It was used by native Americans for asthma, for earaches, toothaches, fatigue, and scores of other afflictions. Smoking was prescribed for things that it very plainly makes worse, not better. Smoking for asthma? Smoking makes asthma worse.

When Europeans made contact with the people of the Americas in the late 1400's, the alleged medicinal value of tobacco was what impressed them about the herb. It wasn't long before smoking and other forms of tobacco consumption were widely prescribed throughout Europe by doctors. It was even widely touted as a panacea, a cure-all.

Why did native Americans and Europeans alike tout tobacco as having such amazing medicinal value? It's a kind of thousands-year-old perfect storm of reasons.

The relief addicts get from smoking provides a convincing illusion that they feel a lot better when they smoke, whatever is ailing them—as long as the smoking is not making them feel lousy, which happens more, over time. In European culture, there is the added capitalist incentive of selling something to people that is addictive. Tell them that it's highly medicinal as a means of attracting and keeping customers.

But, above all, above the physical addiction and the craven force of jackals anxious to exploit weakness, there is the human desire to be comforted with medicine from our afflictions. We are sometimes afraid and seek something to bolster us. Life is challenging and we feel we need help with the challenges we face, often. Psychological addiction is all about believing we are getting crucial help from something that isn't helping us at all—on the contrary, it's hurting us, but we attribute to it the ability to help us get through what we need to get through. The idea that it's hurting us, not helping us, seems ridiculous because we plainly need help and can't do it without some help. Yet we *do* do it without help, have been doing it without help all this time. On our own. The addiction has merely served to provide the illusion of help—and to poison us.

From now until the end of the world—and from now back in time to the dawn of consciousness—we have felt insecure and inadequate to the tasks in front of us, to survive and make our way in the world. We have felt fear and looked for help for our fear and for our limitations. That's just part of being human. It's not a sin. It's not contemptible. It's an occasional part of being a sentient being.

We are often willing to accept a convincing illusion that something (or someone) is helping us because we so desperately believe we need help and can't make it without some help.

Anyway, this is why that mountain is so high. People want to believe smoking helps them. Smoking has been ascribed any number of medicinal properties that it doesn't have. And those stories go back in western culture to the 1500s and, before that, thousands of years in native American culture. It's the enduring nature of human frailty that gives them their long-livedness, not any enduring medicinal value of tobacco. At best, tobacco provides a comforting illusion of supplying well-being by providing relief from the irritating withdrawal symptoms it itself causes.

There is a very long list of ailments smoking has been said to help with, which it doesn't. There are also many myths about how excruciatingly difficult it is to stop smoking. The former serve to draw you in to smoking and the latter serve to keep you smoking.

It isn't difficult to stop smoking if you dismantle the amplifier of nicotine hunger; you then do not have to exercise outrageous amounts of willpower. The amount of willpower you have to exercise is like the willpower involved in deciding not to cross the street if you don't want to. If you have no desire to cross the street, very little willpower is required to refrain from it.

Western culture has 500+ years of persuasions to smoke, from alleged medicinal powers to intellect-enhancing powers to claims that it makes you sexy or it makes you one of the boys (or girls) or it just plain feels good...you would think there's virtually nothing it can't help you with, to judge from the claims made for it over the years.

Governments have had an interest in people smoking because of the tax revenues it brings in. Health-care has been involved first by using smoking as something that was prescribed for many ailments and then, later, in developing the whole apparatus to treat the ailments caused by smoking. Medicine now has a different approach: help people stop smoking by transferring their addiction to gums and other nicotine replacements. This merely transfers their addiction to a product controlled by the health care system. You pay them (and the government, still) rather than the tobacco companies.

Dismantling the psychological addiction is not difficult, but it relinquishes the customer. It sets the addict free from her/his addiction and from financial dependence on the nicotine supplier. It frees the consumer from being consumed by the businesses feeding on them. It *gives* addicts something rather than *taking* from them, *exploiting* them.

Obviously it's much less profitable than selling addicts their ongoing fix. But for anyone who has lost loved ones to lung cancer or throat cancer or any number of other smoking-related diseases, there is no sweeter gift you can give someone than to help them grasp and take their freedom from nicotine addiction. That freedom doesn't solve all your problems in life, but it solves a bunch of them.

And, if you want it to last, which of course you do, you have to cultivate your joy. Every time you feel the dying twinges of desire for a cigarette, which will only happen for about a week, and those twinges won't be very strong at all—not anywhere near an 'urge'— you must rejoice in your freedom from smoking. You may observe the twinge of mild hunger you are feeling and regard it as a specimen, as a little dying monster in a test tube. The little monster would be pitiable were it not such a vile blood-sucker indifferent to your destruction. Soon to be dead after a week when your physical addiction is over.

Feel the joy of knowing that you are free from 'urges' to smoke. Relish it. Think about what it is that freed you: your understanding that smoking does not give you what you thought it gave you. And you can't so easily fool yourself into it any more than you can fall for a card trick you understand the workings of.

Also, something else that's very important to understand about what freed you: you might not realize it or give yourself much credit for it but it's very important. *You were brave.* You opened your eyes and looked at something you've been studiously ignoring. You looked carefully at why you continued to smoke and you looked at whether it was giving you what you thought it was giving you and you realized and acknowledged that it wasn't.

You have dismantled your psychological addiction to smoking which amplified the twinge of mild hunger into 'urges' to smoke. You have dismantled the amplifier. And have begun to build a different amplifier. An amplifier of your joy and freedom into something that helps you appreciate your freedom and know it to be something you don't want to surrender.

That is important to keeping your freedom. Every time you get a twinge to have a cigarette, ask yourself if it's a twinge or an urge. It should just be a twinge, a small twitch of a dying physical addiction, if this book is working for you. If this book is working for you, when you get such mindless small twitches, which you will, occasionally, for about a week, consider it simply as a reminder for you to appreciate your new found freedom, health, and awareness. If you didn't know already, you have come to understand what it means to free yourself from powerful illusions. That's a strong experience that you can accomplish in various spheres. Like what? What other illusions on other matters do we cherish?[31]

You've attained a new perspective not only on smoking and stopping smoking, but on yourself, desire and illusion, freedom and slavery, corporate conformity and personal choice.

Some methods of stopping smoking would have you do things like count your blessings while you still really want a cigarette. That's not the idea here. The whole idea is to get you to a point where you don't have any desire for a cigarette whatsoever. At the start of the book, I said that what I need from you is a commitment to stop smoking if, by the end of the book, you weren't experiencing urges to smoke. If you have reached that point, you can hardly deny your knowledge that the addiction is primarily psychological and that you have the key to your freedom in your hand. You understand it. Cultivate that knowledge. Use it to free yourself and others.

Remember that you're hooked when you think you want one. You have to be honest with yourself and ask yourself if it's a twitch or an urge. If it's a twitch, then it will pass very quickly. It's simply a dying physical addiction. If it's an urge, then the amplifier is working. It means you are still hooked. Where is the hook set? What do you think smoking gives you? Give the book another read. If you haven't read Allen Carr's book *The Easy Way to Stop Smoking*, read it.

If the book isn't working for you, that is, if you are not going to stop smoking now, that's OK. It doesn't work for everyone, but most

---

31 See the Robert Kenner documentary *Merchants of Doubt* that links tobacco companies' efforts to cast doubt on the health risks of smoking and oil companies' efforts to cast doubt on the science of climate change. The documentary was inspired by the book of the same name by historians of science Naomi Oreskes and Erik Conway.

people at least learn important things that will help them permanently stop—eventually. If it isn't working for you, the important thing is to move on without blaming yourself. Try another method that appeals to you as soon as possible. For many people, stopping smoking requires a bit of practice. But if your attitude has changed—if you are no longer OK with remaining hooked indefinitely—then you are on the road to freedom, *and you will succeed*. Because your desire to be free of it is the main thing that will take you there. You may feel powerless to stop, but your desire to stop is very powerful, even if it seems small to you. It will eventually triumph as surely as day follows night. It may seem like you have made no progress toward stopping, but that is not the case. You have to learn how to deal with the things we've discussed. Perhaps most importantly, you need to be able to banish fear enough to keep on trying.

It's been one of the most important things in my life to stop smoking and then to write this book to hopefully help others do the same. I hope it helps you attain a new perspective not only on smoking but on the related issues we've talked about throughout the book. And that reading this book helps you to stop smoking permanently. Thank you for reading the book; best wishes to you.

You are a seeker of truth and freedom. Who would unknow anything of what they now know? No one who seeks and values the truth. Who would love the chains of their enslavement? No one who knows they hold the key. Cast off your chains and walk free.

61 - Bibliography

- *The Easy Way to Stop Smoking*, Allen Carr, Arcturus Publishing, 1985

- *Tobacco and Shamanism in South America*, Johannes Wilbert, Yale University Press, 1987

- *Tobacco Use by Native North Americans*, Joseph C. Winter (ed), University of Oklahoma Press, 2000

- *Tobacco in History – The Cultures of Dependence*, Jordan Goodman, Routledge, London, 1993

- *In the Realm of Hungry Ghosts: Close Encounters with Addiction*, Gabor Maté, Knopf Canada, 2009

- *Smoke: A Global History of Smoking*, Sander L. Gilman and Zhou Xun (ed), Reaktion Books, London, 2004

- *Narcotic Culture: A History of Drugs in China*, Frank Dikötter, Lars Laamann, Zhou Xun, University of Chicago Press, 2004

- *Merchants of Doubt*, Naomi Oreskes and Erik M. Conway (2010 book), Robert Kenner (2014 video)

- What Is Addiction? (3:24 video) Gabor Maté on the nature of addiction: filmsforaction.org/watch/what-is-addiction-gabor-mate

- *Salt Sugar Fat — How the Food Giants Hooked Us*, Michael Moss, Penguin Random House, 2013

- Smoker face: A brief overview of capnolagnia: drmarkgriffiths.wordpress.com/2012/10/23/smoker-face-a-brief-overview-of-capnolagnia

- Hočąk (Winnebago) tobacco origin myth: hotcakencyclopedia.com/ho.TobaccoOriginMyth.html

- Royal College of Psychiatrists: It's time to support older people in giving up smoking: rcpsych.ac.uk/mediacentre/pressreleases2015/olderpeopleandsmoking.aspx

- Centers for Disease Control and Prevention: cdc.gov/tobacco

Lightning Source UK Ltd.
Milton Keynes UK
UKOW02f1536291116

288799UK00001B/112/P

9 780994 953100